Imaging in Critical Care Medicine

Imaging in critically ill patients is a ubiquitous but challenging line of investigation for the physician as accurate interpretation is often difficult as patient cooperation during the procedure is grossly compromised, and the resultant image is often suboptimal. This book provides details on principles of imaging and the diagnostic hallmarks of common diseases to assist in correct interpretation. It contains guidance to overcome the deficiencies observed during the performance of bedside imaging and equipment handling and addresses the rationale for various procedural/management and imaging approaches. This is a useful companion for most doctors and trainees working in critical care settings.

Key Features

- Features case-based scenarios in critical care as well as a section on tropical diseases
- Appeals to a wide audience of trainees and consultants of critical care medicine, internal medicine, anaesthesiology, pulmonary medicine and those working in the ICU, due to its clinical relevance
- Reduces the dependency on the radiologist and helps physician save time, enhancing the quality of patient care

Imaging in Critical Care Medicine

Edited by

Anirban Hom Choudhuri
Director Professor (Critical Care)
Department of Anesthesiology & Intensive Care
GIPMER, New Delhi, India

Ashish Verma
Professor & Head
Department of Radio Diagnosis & Intervention Radiology
Institute of Medical Sciences, BHU
Varanasi, Uttar Pradesh, India

Associate Editor: Ishan Kumar
Associate Professor
Department of Radiodiagnosis and Interventional Radiology
Institute of Medical Sciences, Banaras Hindu University
Varanasi, India

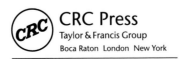

CRC Press
Taylor & Francis Group
Boca Raton London New York

CRC Press is an imprint of the
Taylor & Francis Group, an **informa** business

Cover Image: © Shutterstock images

First edition published 2024
by CRC Press
6000 Broken Sound Parkway NW, Suite 300, Boca Raton, FL 33487–2742

and by CRC Press
4 Park Square, Milton Park, Abingdon, Oxon, OX14 4RN

CRC Press is an imprint of Taylor & Francis Group, LLC

© 2024 selection and editorial matter, Anirban Hom Choudhuri and Ashish Verma;
individual chapters, the contributors

Library of Congress Cataloging-in-Publication Data
Names: Choudhuri, Anirban Hom, editor. | Verma, Ashish (Professor of radiology), editor.
Title: Imaging in critical care medicine / edited by Anirban Hom Choudhuri, Ashish Verma ; associate
    editor, Ishan Kumar
Description: First edition. | Boca Raton, FL : CRC Press, 2023. | Includes bibliographical references and
    index. | Summary: "Imaging in critically ill patients is a ubiquitous but challenging line of investigation
    for the physician as accurate interpretation is often difficult as patient cooperation during the procedure
    is grossly compromised, and the resultant image is often suboptimal. This book provides details on
    principles of imaging and the diagnostic hallmarks of common diseases helping in correct interpretation.
    It contains guidance to overcome the deficiencies observed during the performance of bedside
    imaging and equipment handling and addresses the rationale for various procedural/management and
    imaging approaches. This is a useful companion for most doctors and trainees working in critical care
    settings"—Provided by publisher.
Identifiers: LCCN 2023000930 (print) | LCCN 2023000931 (ebook) | ISBN 9781032111780 (hardback) |
    ISBN 9781032111773 (paperback) | ISBN 9781003218739 (ebook)
Subjects: MESH: Diagnostic Imaging | Critical Care | Critical Illness
Classification: LCC RC78.7.D53 (print) | LCC RC78.7.D53 (ebook) | NLM WN 180 |
    DDC 616.07/54—dc23/eng/20230429
LC record available at https://lccn.loc.gov/2023000930
LC ebook record available at https://lccn.loc.gov/2023000931

ISBN: 978-1-032-11178-0 (hbk)
ISBN: 978-1-032-11177-3 (pbk)
ISBN: 978-1-003-21873-9 (ebk)

DOI: 10.1201/9781003218739

Typeset in Minion Pro
by Apex CoVantage, LLC

Dedication

The book is dedicated to our parents, all our respected teachers and our beloved students.

Contents

Foreword   viii

Preface   ix

Acknowledgments   x

Editors   xi

Contributors   xii

Introduction   xiii

1   Respiratory system   1
    Ashish Verma, Bhuvna Ahuja, Sakshi Duggal and Ishan Kumar
2   Cardiovascular system   28
    *Sandeep Kar, Kakali Ghosh, Pavan Kumar Dallampati and
    Anirban Hom Choudhuri*
3   Nervous system   47
    Ishan Kumar, Ashish Verma and Bhuvna Ahuja
4   Locomotor system   68
    Vaishali Upadhyay, Khushboo Pilania and Anirban Hom Choudhuri
5   Urogenital system   93
    Surabhi Vyas, Smita Manchanda and Anirban Hom Choudhuri
6   Gastrointestinal system   116
    Ashish Verma, Sakshi Duggal and Ishan Kumar
7   The pregnant patient   139
    Smita Manchanda, Surabhi Vyas and Ashish Verma
8   Pediatric imaging   154
    Ishan Kumar, Ashish Verma and Anirban Hom Choudhuri
9   Interventional radiology in critically ill patients   171
    Ranjan Kumar Patel, Tanya Yadav and Amar Mukund

Index   194

Foreword

It is a privilege for me to introduce to readers a versatile compendium entitled, *Imaging in Critical Care Medicine*, a book edited by Professor Anirban Hom Choudhuri and Professor Ashish Verma and published by CRC Press/Taylor & Francis.

Critical Care Medicine is one of the foremost disciplines where imaging has a major role to play for the diagnosis and prognostication of patients. The discipline requires a thorough knowledge of various complex and diverse illnesses where clinical examination in isolation, however good and meticulous, falls short in identifying all the problems. Moreover, the decisions for therapeutic interventions need to be made in very short time spans. Having worked for most of my career in managing critically ill liver disease patients, I know that the clinical assessment of the intensivist often needs a good correlation with the imaging modalities and laboratory tests.

The modern-day intensivists need to learn and interpret the radiological findings with much more precision and expertise than before without becoming dependent totally on the radiologists for their interpretation. This is not to make them substitutes for the radiologists but to ensure that timely therapy is not delayed in critically ill patients. The benefits of timely initiation of therapy are immense and all efforts should be taken to reap these advantages. Moreover, the bedside application of imaging techniques for both diagnosis and therapeutic interventions barring the need for any patient transfer to radiology suite has become a big boon in medical practice. It has also become the norm in many places whenever feasible, and intensivists must be more competent in their execution.

I have known both Professors Choudhuri and Verma for a long time as experts in the field of critical care medicine and radiology, respectively. I appreciate their endeavor to edit this important book, which will be extremely useful for all physicians handling critically ill patients in general and for the practitioners of Critical Care, Emergency Medicine and Anesthesiology, in particular. The contents are rich and cover all the aspects of imaging in critical care that are encountered routinely. Lastly, I applaud the experts that have contributed to enrich this volume, which I do hope will reach the desks of fellows and faculty members of critical care medicine across Asia. My compliments also to CRC Press/Taylor & Francis for undertaking this much needed initiative.

Dr S.K. Sarin
Director, ILBS
New Delhi

Preface

The correct diagnosis of any critical illness is a crucial determinant for its outcome. Even if the disease is advanced and in an irreversible stage, a correct diagnosis can deter unnecessary tests, forbear unwanted admissions and circumvent undesirable medicines, but clinical diagnosis may sometimes be erroneous or flawed. Hence, laboratory and imaging modalities assume immense value to the physicians in such states. This is particularly true for emergency rooms and critical care units.

Choosing an appropriate test from a wide range of available modalities is not so easy. Many factors, such as the time duration required for completing the test, risk of radiation hazards, patients' tolerance to the administration of contrast media etc., determine the final choice. Additionally, the physician is expected to interpret the results correctly without any inordinate delay.

This book will serve as a quick reference to physicians about the significance, rationale and procedural maneuvers for employing different radiological investigations in the emergency room and critical care units. Each chapter incorporates the imaging modalities in serial fashion, starting from the most basic and going up to the most advanced.

Acknowledgments

We express our sincere thanks to all the authors listed in the list of contributors for their valuable contribution in the form of chapters and images.

We acknowledge with thanks the support from Dr Girish MP and Dr Mohit Gupta, both professors in the Cardiology Department of GIPMER, New Delhi, for providing us with valuable images for the textbook.

We thank our publishers, Taylor & Francis/CRC Press, for providing all possible help for the successful and time-bound completion of the book.

We also thank our colleagues, friends and well-wishers for encouraging us to write this book, and last but not the least we acknowledge the immense support from our family members, who continuously supported us and made large sacrifices to allow us the time to devote for this book.

In the end, we hope that readers will appreciate our hard work and give us their valuable feedback to enable us to improve this book further in successive editions.

Editors

Dr Anirban Hom Choudhuri is Director Professor in the Critical Care Division of the Department of Anesthesia & Intensive Care at GB Pant Institute of Post Graduate Medical Education and Research, New Delhi. He has also worked previously at AIIMS New Delhi, Tata Memorial Centre, Mumbai and Escort Heart Institute & Research Centre, New Delhi. He has authored numerous original research articles, textbook chapters and meta-analyses in various journals of critical care and is also the reviewer in many more. He is on the expert committees of many regulatory bodies and examiner in five universities in critical care medicine.

Dr Ashish Verma is the Professor and Head of Diagnostic and Intervention Radiology in the Institute of Medical Sciences, BHU Varanasi. He has also worked previously at SGPGIMS Lucknow, ILBS New Delhi and Tata Memorial Center, Mumbai. He is the author in various journals, textbooks, and so on, and a regular examiner at eminent institutes and universities. He is a part of the expert committee in some international societies in interventional radiology.

Contributors

Bhuvna Ahuja
Assistant Professor
(Neuroanesthesia)
LNJP & MAMC
New Delhi, India

Anirban Hom Choudhuri
Director Professor (Critical Care)
Department of Anesthesiology &
Intensive Care
GIPMER
New Delhi, India

Pavan Kumar Dallampati
DM Trainee
(Cardiac Anesthesia)
IPGMER
Kolkata, West Bengal, India

Sakshi Duggal
Assistant Professor
(Anesthesia & Intensive Care)
ESIC Medical College
Basaidarapur, New Delhi,
India

Kakali Ghosh
Associate Professor
(Cardiac Anesthesia)
IPGMER
Kolkata, West Bengal, India

Sandeep Kar
Assistant Professor
(Cardiac Anesthesia)
IPGMER
Kolkata, West Bengal,
India

Ishan Kumar
Associate Professor
Department of Radio Diagnosis &
Intervention Radiology
Institute of Medical Sciences, BHU
Varanasi, Uttar Pradesh, India

Smita Manchanda
Additional Professor
Department of Radio Diagnosis &
Intervention Radiology
AIIMS
New Delhi, India

Khushboo Pilania
Consultant (Radiology)
Izen Imaging & Interventions
Noida, Uttar Pradesh, India

Vaishali Upadhyaya
Consultant (Radiology)
Vivekananda Polyclinic & Institute
of Medical Sciences
Lucknow, Uttar Pradesh, India

Ashish Verma
Professor and Head
Department of Radio Diagnosis &
Intervention Radiology
Institute of Medical Sciences, BHU
Varanasi, Uttar Pradesh, India

Surabhi Vyas
Additional Professor
Department of Radio Diagnosis &
Intervention Radiology
AIIMS
New Delhi, India

Introduction

The intensive care unit is a place where many investigations are routinely performed from time to time. Among them, a major share is borne by the radiological image. The investigations vary from the most basic such as the X-ray and ultrasonography to the most advanced such as MRI. While some investigations are undertaken for diagnostic purposes, many are also performed with the aim of intervention.

The literature is scant about the usefulness of various imaging modalities in the ICU during the course of various illnesses. The intensivists need proper training and guidance to help them advise radiological images and also interpret the results scientifically. This textbook should prove useful as a ready-made source of practical information at such times.

Each chapter has been divided section-wise to highlight the cardinal pointers and diagnostic hallmarks. The differential diagnosis has been also discussed vividly. Some of the illustrations have been adapted for better understanding in a format similar to the international fellowship exams.

Respiratory system

ASHISH VERMA, BHUVNA AHUJA,
SAKSHI DUGGAL AND ISHAN KUMAR

INTRODUCTION

Respiratory imaging is the most frequently performed radiological investigation in the ICU. It is undertaken in patients with respiratory diseases, cardiac disorders, neurological illnesses etc. Since many patients in the ICU are unable to narrate their history and symptoms, their interpretation requires correlation with the clinical signs. They are not only important for the sake of diagnosis but also to monitor the course of illness in the ICU and prognosticate the outcomes.

AIM OF IMAGING

a. To look for features that may directly explain the symptoms, e.g. a patch of consolidation in a patient with fever
b. To confirm diagnosis in the presence of multiple provisional diagnoses, e.g. tell-tale sign of pulmonary tuberculosis in a case with acute abdomen suspected due to abdominal tuberculosis
c. To detect additional findings on the basis of presumption from underlying aetiology, e.g. extrapulmonary thoracic fluid suggesting hemothorax in a patient of polytrauma
d. To ensure safety during the conduct of any emergency intervention under anaesthesia

DOI: 10.1201/9781003218739-1

IMAGING MODALITIES

The key modalities that are useful in everyday practice include:

- **Chest X-ray**
  - Best taken in upright PA or AP position; lateral decubitus views are useful in the presence of minimal pleural fluid
  - Supine AP views are evaluated with caution as many structures look different, e.g. heart appears larger, fluid level is not appreciated in the horizontal plane
  - Good for initial screening
  - Helps in comparing right and left thoracic cavities
  - Useful for detecting pneumothorax and/or pleural effusion, as also pneumoperitoneum (in PA view)
  - Detects fractures and bony deformities

- **Ultrasonography**
  - Can be performed in any position
  - Often combined with chest X-ray
  - Performed using a high-frequency (5–20 Mhz) linear electronic array transducer/probe with small imaging head. High-frequency micro-convex probes are also used
  - Useful in detecting free fluid in thorax (though not ideal for detecting free air)
  - Possible to evaluate abdomen and heart alongside lungs
  - Identifies abnormalities in soft tissues, viscera and blood vessels (but not bones)
  - Differentiates pleural effusion from thickening
  - Differentiates exudative (slightly echogenic) from transudative (totally anechoic) effusion
  - Acts as a guide for placement of central lines, chest tubes etc.
  - May be repeated multiple times as there are no risks of radiation hazard

- **CT Scan**
  - Detecting underlying malignancies
  - Diagnosing the presence of pleural thickening (and characterizing the same) or bronchopleural fistula along with effusion
  - Ruling out any interstitial lung disease, pulmonary embolism

- **Other Investigations**
  - Ventilation perfusion (VQ) scan: diagnosis of pulmonary embolism (except in the acute phase)

CARDINAL TECHNICAL POINTERS

- **Pneumothorax**
  - *Chest X-ray*
    - Use upright films (sitting or semi-recline if not possible)
    - Expiratory film is preferred and may be achieved by observing the breathing pattern for a patient not on ventilator

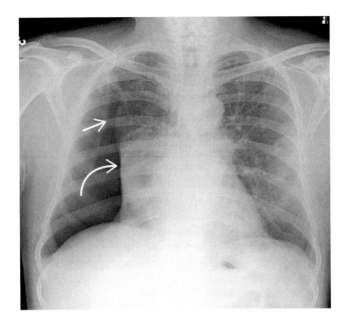

Figure 1.1 Chest radiograph frontal view in supine AP position shows hyperlucency without broncho-vascular markings suggestive of air (*white arrow*) in the right pleural cavity with volume loss of right lung; as a result the right lung (*curved white arrow*) has partially collapsed s/o pneumothorax causing compressive atelectasis. The outline of the collapsed lung is seen well against the air.

- Sensitivity: 39–52%; Specificity: 99–100%
- Diagnostic sign: hyperlucent areas in thorax; absence of bronchovascular markings within these hyperlucent areas
- USG
  - Best obtained in supine or lateral decubitus (diseased side up) position
  - Sensitivity 78–90%; Specificity > 98%
  - Diagnostic sign: absent lung sliding (negative predictive value: 100%); absent B-lines; lung point (specific for pneumothorax, shows air-air interface); seashore with stratosphere signs; double lung point (M-mode showing interleaved waveforms for sliding and non-sliding lung at the two opposite sides of the same scan; hydro-point (specific for hydropneumothorax and shows air-fluid interface)
- Assessment criteria
  - Collins method – % = 4.2 + 4.7 (maximum apical interpleural distance + interpleural distance at midpoint of upper half of lung + interpleural distance at midpoint of lower half of lung)
  - Other less commonly used methods: Rhea method, light index

- **Pleural effusion (Figure 1.2)**
  - *Chest X-ray*
    - Upright films are the best (sitting or semi-recline if not possible), especially if associated with pneumothorax; supine films can be taken when patients cannot sit or recline
    - Best detected in inspiratory phase
    - Sensitivity: 24–100%; Specificity: 85–100%
    - Diagnostic sign: focal or diffuse haziness or increased opacity in hemithorax (in supine AP view if fluid spreads; also in PA view if effusion is minimal and rises up due to capillary action); fluid meniscus (if no air associated) or fluid level if air associated with fluid; blunting of costophrenic/cardio-phrenic angles; elliptical homogenous mass of fluid density (if effusion is loculated in any focal region between two pleural layers); secondary mass effect on adjacent structures such as mediastinum; sub-pulmonic/infra-pulmonic effusion is seen as raised hemidiaphragm or increased liver span superiorly on right side and increased distance between gastric bubble and lower lung margin on left side

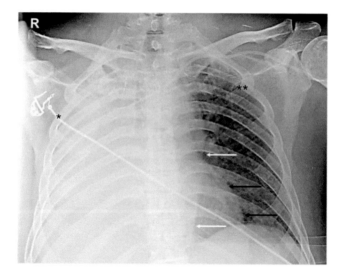

Figure 1.2 Chest radiograph frontal view in erect AP position showing complete 'whiteout' of the right hemithorax. The right cardio-mediastinal silhouette as well as the right hemidiaphragm outline are not visualized. Note that there are no signs of 'net volume gain', such as no widening of the intercostal spaces or shift of the mediastinal structures towards the opposite side. The outline of descending aorta (*straight white arrow*) and that of the left ventricle (*straight black arrow*) are at the expected sites. This indicates towards a massive pleural effusion with collapse of lung. The volume gain caused due to effusion has been compensated by volume loss due to collapse causing no 'net volume gain'. The central venous catheter placed from the left subclavian vein (**) has its tip placed at a position higher than desirable location viz. cavo-atrial junction. The other device seen (*) is an EC lead. The left lung is normal.

- *USG*
  - Best in sitting/semi-recline position or lateral decubitus (diseased side up) position
  - Best site to look for minimal effusion: posterior costophrenic angle after keeping the patient upright for 15 minutes
  - Sensitivity: 92–96%; Specificity: 88–100%
  - Diagnostic sign: echo-free space; quad sign (rectangular anechoic space between parietal pleura–chest wall near the probe, two rib shadows on either side and visceral pleura–lung surface complex known as 'lung line' at the bottom of screen); sinusoid signs (due to movement of visceral pleura on M-mode; may be absent in thick/viscous exudative effusion); fluid color (color signal due to movement of fluid on color Doppler); thoracic spine sign (a bright line with multiple scallops and posterior acoustic shadowing extending beyond the diaphragm); jellyfish sign (lung floating in massive effusion); plankton sign (echogenic floaters/septations representing transudative/complex effusion); hematocrit sign (if patient upright and still for some time a fluid-fluid level forms between fluids of two densities indicative of hemothorax)
- Least amount of fluid that can be detected in X-ray is 50 mL (radiography) and 3–5 mL (sonography): > 20 mL detected with high sensitivity (but this depends a lot on location of fluid also) and ≥ 100 mL with 100% Sn on sonography
- Assessment of fluid volume on USG
  - Balik's formula: patient supine full inspiration, probe perpendicular to posterolateral chest wall; volume in mL = vertical distance between two pleural lines in mm × 20
  - Eibenberger's formula: patient supine full inspiration, probe perpendicular to posterolateral chest wall; volume in mL = 47.6 × distance in cm between the lung and posterior chest wall – 837
  - Goecke's formula: patient upright full expiration, probe perpendicular to posterolateral chest wall; volume in mL = craniocaudal distance between lung and diaphragm in cm × 90

- **Rib fracture**
  - Best to do a CT scan of thorax with 3D reconstructions
  - *X-ray*
    - Use upright films (sitting or semi-recline if standing not possible)
    - AP films are better to evaluate the ribs
  - *USG*
    - Use a liner transducer of 5–10 Mhz
    - Discontinuity of the rib line on longitudinal scan with/without minimal adjacent pleural fluid are usually seen

- **Consolidation and/or collapse (Figure 1.3)**
  - *X-ray*
    - Use upright films (sitting or semi-recline if standing not possible)
    - Inspiratory film is best
    - Diagnostic sign: seen as an opaque area in the otherwise aerated lung

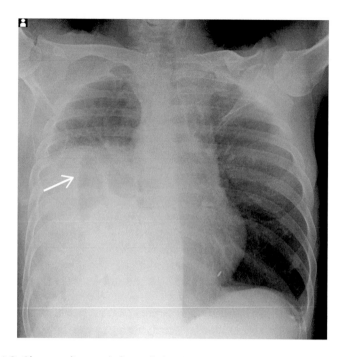

Figure 1.3 Chest radiograph frontal view in supine AP position showing homogeneous confluent opacity in right middle and lower lobes with obscuration of right cardiac border and right hemidiaphragm, some proximal air bronchograms (*white arrow*) s/o right middle and lower lobar consolidation.

- USG
  - Use a liner transducer of 5–10 Mhz; deeper areas of lung may be better seen with a convex low-frequency probe (3–5 Mhz)
  - Best to scan in supine or lateral decubitus (suspected side up) position
  - Approximately 98% consolidations are subpulmonic; hence their presence is revealed during USG evaluation!
  - Diagnostic sign: shred sign (non-translobar consolidation); tissue-like sign (translobar consolidation). Both are 90% sensitive and 98% specific. Other signs are dynamic air–bronchogram sign and lung pulse sign (can also differentiate consolidation from collapse)

- **Phrenic nerve injury and/or diaphragmatic rupture**
  - USG
    - Are usually seen from the abdominal window using low-frequency probe
    - Phrenic palsy is seen as a paradoxical movement of diaphragm with respiration, as one would expect in fluoroscopy

– Diaphragmatic rupture is seen as discontinuity in the echogenic line formed by the lung base diaphragm interface. Associated focal herniation of liver (on right) and spleen (on left) may also be seen

- **Interstitial syndrome**
  - *USG*
    - Represented by lung rockets ($\geq$ 3 B-lines) and is an early manifestation of any disease causing interstitial edema. B-line is always a comet-tail artifact, always arises from the pleural line, and always moves in concert with lung-sliding. It is almost always long, well-defined, laser-like, hyperechoic, erasing A-lines. B1, B2 lines represent advancing patterns of edema leading to alveolar edema

TUBES AND LINES: POSITIONS AND MALPOSITIONS

- *Nasogastric/Orogastric tube (NGT/OGT)*
  - Larger, side-holes
  - Tip anywhere in stomach ($\geq$10 cm) distal to the gastro-esophageal junction, hence seen below the left hemidiaphragm (unless situs inversus); point downward towards the midline; no radio-opaque tip

- *Dobhoff tube (DHT)*
  - Thinner, no side-holes
  - Tip placed in antro-pyloric region; cross the midline; below the right hemidiaphragm; point upward away from midline; radio-opaque tip

- *Endotracheal tube (ETT)*
  - Tip placed approximately 5 cm above carina viz. between medial ends of clavicles above manubrium sternii

- *Central venous catheter (CVC)*
  - Tip should be at the cavo-atrial junction usually located at the first anterior intercostal space towards right of sternal margin
  - In most patients cavo-atrial angle may be seen in the right mediastinal silhouette (viz. straight line of vena cava and outward bulge of right atrium)

- *Intercostal drain (ICD)*
  - Tip should be evaluated on two views (AP and lateral)
  - Unless placed in a loculated effusion (when it is located at the effusion site), it should point upwards and located at posterior or lateral costophrenic angle

- *Permanent pacemaker (PPM)*
  - Tip of the electrode should be in the right atrial appendage (atrial pacing) or right ventricular apex (ventricular pacing). In case of double chamber pacing, both may be seen
  - Tip fracture common and may be searched for

- *Thermometer probe*
  - Tip located in esophagus up till D7. Lateral view may also be needed to confirm

- *Pericardial drain*
  - Tip on the left of midline into the pericardial space. Lateral view may also be needed to confirm

- *Intra-aortic balloon pump (IABP)*
  - Tip at the level of the aortopulmonary window. Lateral view may also be needed to confirm

READING A CHEST X-RAY

Step I: Quality assessment of the radiograph (Figure 1.4)
First ensure that the X-ray is of correct patient, and Left/Right has been correctly marked.

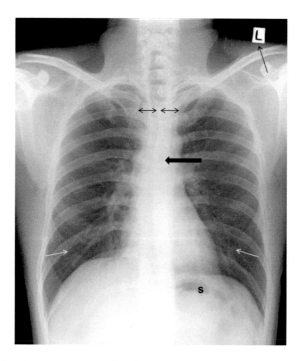

Figure 1.4 Quality assessment of radiograph. Chest X-ray PA view image showing (a) left side has been correctly marked (*black arrow*); (b) exposure quality is adequate, suggested by faint visibility of vertebrae behind the heart (*solid black arrow*); (c) adequate inspiratory effort is evident by visualization of anterior sixth ribs (*white arrows*); (d) non-rotation as the spinoud process is equidistant from the medial end of clavicles (*double arrows*); and the radiograph taken in erect posture suggested by visualization of gastric fundus air(s).

- *Exposure quality*: adequate penetration is said when the vertebral bodies are faintly visible through the heart.
- *View and posture*: ask the nurse/X-ray technician whether it is AP/PA view, also whether X-ray has been performed in supine/erect posture. Heart and mediastinal structures are subject to magnification on AP view and thus may lead to false interpretation of cardiomegaly.
- *Patient rotation*: the medial ends of both clavicles should be equidistant from the spinous process of the vertebra between the clavicle. If not so, patient would be rotated during X-ray exposure and may lead to unilateral enlargement of cardiomediastinal contour. Also, there is increase in blackness of the hemi-thorax on the side to which the patient is rotated.
- *Adequacy of inspiratory effort*: six complete anterior or ten posterior ribs should be visible.

Step II: Anatomical structures to be evaluated (Figure 1.5)
1. *Trachea and bronchi*
   a. Trachea is a midline radiolucent structure, which might be slightly deviated to the right side at the level of the aortic arch. It divides into a short right main bronchus and a longer and more horizontal left main bronchus.
   b. Try to look for abrupt cut-off or localized narrowing of trachea.

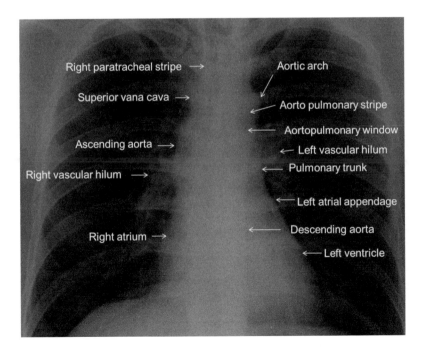

Figure 1.5 Normal chest radiograph PA view showing the structures outlining the cardiomediastinal contour.

    c. In case of deviated trachea, try to determine if it is pulled or pushed. Trachea can be pulled towards atelectatic lung. Space-occupying lesions in paratracheal locations/upper mediastinum can push the trachea.

    d. Evaluate subcarinal angle (>1000), can be due to left atrial enlargement, pericardial effusion or subcarinal masses.

2. *Upper mediastinum*

    a. First assess the right and left paratracheal stripe.

    b. On the right side of trachea, there is a right paratracheal stripe extending from clavicle to tracheobronchial angle. This stripe is <4mm thick, and a thickened right paratracheal stripe may be due to paratracheal lymph nodes, pleural effusion, thyroid, parathyroid or tracheal wall lesions.

    c. Left paratracheal stripe is formed by the intervening soft tissues between the trachea and left upper lobe. Widened left paratracheal stripe can be due to lymph nodes or thyroid/parathyroid masses.

    d. Aortopulmonary stripe is formed by anterior mediastinal fat and left upper lobe anterior to aortic arch and left pulmonary artery seen as a straight line crossing the aortic arch. Anterior mediastinal mass can lead to obliterated stripe or convex AP stripe towards left lung. Pneumomediastinum can elevate the stripe.

    e. Try to evaluate two convex bulges on left side, which is formed by aortic knob and pulmonary trunk. Aortopulmonary window lies posterior to the aortopulmonary stripe, extending from inferior wall of the aortic arch to superior wall of the left pulmonary artery. It is usually concave or sometimes straight, and its convex contour of the AP window is considered abnormal and may be due to tumors, lymph nodes or bronchial artery aneurysm.

    f. Widened mediastinum is diagnosed if mediastinal width is greater than 6 cm on an upright PA chest X-ray or 8 cm on supine AP chest film. Causes of widened mediastinum are thoracic aortic aneurysms or congenital heart and great vessel disease as well as lymph nodal and mediastinal masses.

3. *Cardiac silhouette* (Figure 1.6)

    a. First, evaluate for cardiomegaly. A cardiothoracic ratio (CTR) >50% on PA view is considered as a sign of cardiomegaly. It should be noted that this sign is 80% specific and 50% sensitive for left ventricular enlargement.

    b. Increased CTR and shifting of apex towards left side are signs of left ventricular enlargement.

    c. Shifting of apex upwards and to the left are signs of right ventricular enlargement.

    d. Next, carefully assess the cardiomediastinal contour. The left contour is formed by aortic arch, pulmonary trunk, left atrial appendage and left ventricle (superior to inferior). The right contour is formed by SVC, right atrium and sometimes IVC.

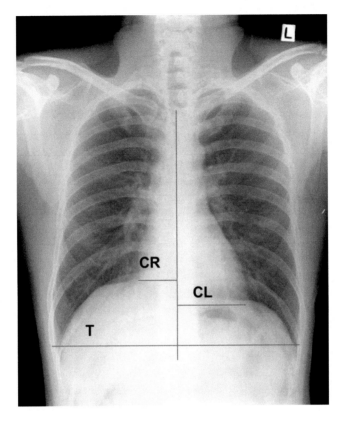

Figure 1.6 Cardiothoracic radio. The ratio (CR+CL)/T more than 0.5 is suggestive of cardiomegaly.

   e. Straightening of left heart border, elevation of left bronchus with wide subcarinal angle, and bulging/double right border are signs of left atrial enlargement (most commonly due to mitral valve disease). Focal convexity below left bronchus is a sign of left atrial appendage enlargement.

4. *Hilar structures*

   a. Hila connect the lungs to mediastinum and are formed by superior pulmonary veins and lower pulmonary arteries. Point of intersection (hilar point) forms concave angles bilaterally. Left hilum is usually superior to right.

   b. Increased size and density of hilum, convex hilar angle, obscured interlobar artery and lobulated contour of vessels hilar can be due to hilar lymph nodes.

   c. Hilum overlay sign: masses anterior or posterior to hilar vessels result in hilar opacity, but the margins of the hilar vessels are clearly demarcated.

d. Prominent vessels: RPDA >16 mm and LDPA >18 mm are suggestive of pulmonary hypertension.

e. Increased caliber of upper lobe pulmonary veins compared to lower lobe vessels (cephalization/stag antler's sign) can be seen in pulmonary edema. The measurement should be made in vessels at equal distance from the hilar point.

f. If a hilum has moved, you should try to determine if it has been pushed or pulled, just as you would for the trachea. Ask yourself if there is a lung abnormality that has reduced volume of one hemithorax (pulled), or if there has been increase in volume or pressure of the other hemithorax (pushed).

5. *Lungs* (Figures 1.7 and 1.8)

a. Lungs are divided into zones while describing a pathology on frontal radiographs because middle lobe and lingular segment are located anterior to lower lobes.

The lung zones are arbitrarily defined as:

   i. Apical zone: above clavicle
   ii. Upper zone from the apex to 2nd costal cartilage
   iii. Mid-zone: between 2nd and 4th costal cartilage
   iv. Lower zone: below 4th costal cartilage

b. There are four patterns of opacities seen in lungs:

   i. Consolidation: lobar, segmental, diffuse or multifocal. Try to ascertain its location based on silhouette sign.
   ii. Atelectasis (collapse): sharply defined opacity obscuring vessels without air-bronchogram associated with volume loss resulting in

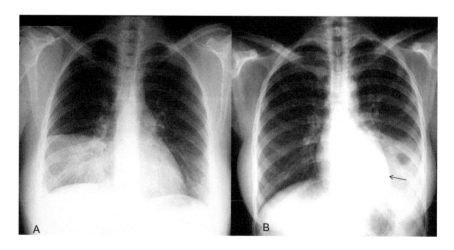

Figure 1.7 Consolidation and silhouette sign. (A) Middle lobe consolidation: lobar consolidation in right lower 'zone' indistinct right heart border suggests anterior location of consolidation in vicinity of heart. (B) Lower lobe consolidation: consolidation in left lower 'zone' with well-visualized left heart border (*arrow*), which suggests that consolidation is posteriorly located not close to heart.

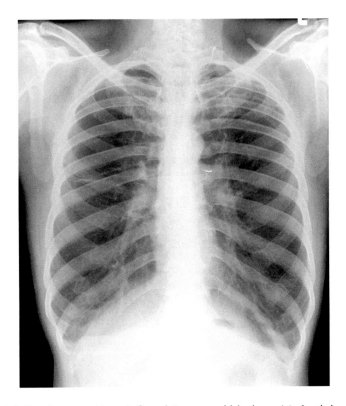

Figure 1.8 Emphysema. Hyperinflated (increased blackness) in both lungs with flatted bilateral diaphragms, blunted CP angles and visualization of more than six anterior ribs.

   displacement of diaphragm, fissures, hili or mediastinum towards the opacity.
  iii. Nodules/masses.
  iv. Interstitial pattern: (reticular or reticulonodular opacities).
 c. It should be noted that categorization of the lung findings into these patterns is not always possible.
 d. Comparison with previous X-rays should be made.
6. *Costophrenic angles and pleura* (Figures 1.9 and 1.10)
 a. Pleural effusion can be visible as blunting of costophrenic angle or lung base opacities obscuring CP angle, a C-shaped meniscus is formed in erect posture. It takes 200 mL of pleural fluid to be visualized on X-ray.
 b. Fluid entrapped within fissures can be seen as well-defined rounded opacities (vanishing tumor). Loculated pleural effusions can be identified using:
  i. Incomplete border sign (well-defined opacity along the chest wall with inner well-defined border and ill-defined outer border merging with chest wall) and

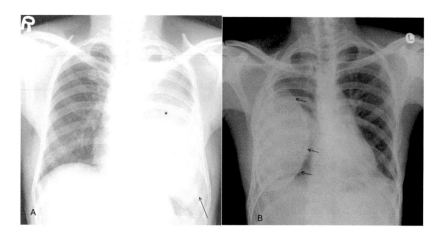

Figure 1.9 Pleural effusion (A) asymmetric opacity in left hemithorax (*) with obscured left CP angle (*long arrow*) and (B) loculated opacity along right chest wall with margins (*arrows*) forming obtuse angle with heart in a case of right-sided empyema.

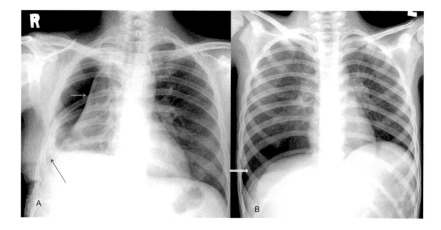

Figure 1.10 (A) Right-sided pleural air collection with clearly visible lung outline (*white arrow*) along with blunting of right CP angle with an opacity forming meniscus, suggestive of right hydropneumothorax and (B) X-ray in supine position (absent gastric fundus air) showing deep right CP angle with localized blackness and absence of lung markings, suggestive of right pneumothorax.

      ii. Extrapleural sign (lesions having oblique margins that taper slowly to the chest wall forming obtuse angle).

   c. Pneumothorax can be identified by visualization of retracted visceral pleura (straight line) and absence of vascular markings lateral to that.

In supine position, lucent and deep cardiophrenic angle (deep sulcus sign) can be seen in pneumothorax.

7. *Diaphragm*: right hemidiaphragm is seen superior to left hemidiaphragm. Left diaphragm is partially obscured due to heart shadow. Complete visualization of left diaphragm is a sign of pneumomediastinum (continuous diaphragm sign).

8. *Bones*
   a. Careful scrutiny of all the ribs (anterior to posterior), vertebrae, scapula, clavicles and the shoulder joints should be done.
   b. Bilateral paraspinal regions should be evaluated, especially the areas obscured by the heart, for presence of any added opacity.

9. *Soft tissue* should be evaluated for asymmetry, breast lesions, gastric fundus air and visualized neck.

10. *Care must be taken* to evaluate the hidden areas of thorax once again:
    a. Lung apices
    b. 'Behind' the heart
    c. Under the diaphragm

11. *Location of tubes and lines* should be confirmed, such as pleural/pericardial drainage tube, endotracheal tube, nasogastric tube, central line etc.

FREQUENTLY ASKED QUESTIONS

- **Difference between computerized radiography (CR) and digital radiography (DR):** Both of these are advanced forms of radiography where, instead of a radiographic film in a cassette, we use an imaging plate (in CR) or a detector plate (in DR). In a CR, the imaging plate (IP) has to be read in a CR reader, during which process the information gathered during exposure is erased and the IP becomes ready for another exposure. In a DR, the detector is directly connected to the computer system via infrared or Bluetooth connectivity, such that as soon as the exposure of X-ray is done, the image appears on the computer screen. Both of these modalities offer the facility to manipulate the image contrast if some error in exposure is there. Further soft-copy images are available, which may be transmitted to an expert for reading without any distortion.

- **Gray scale (B-mode), M-mode, color Doppler, pulse wave (PW) and continuous wave (CW) Doppler, spectral Doppler/Doppler flow velocity waveform, duplex Doppler:** The routine sonography that we do is the gray scale or B-mode sonography, which is generated as a result of reflection of the ultrasound beam from various layers of tissues within the part of interest, depending on relative elasticity. Sonographic examination routinely begins with gray-scale evaluation. When the same signal is utilized to form a map of tissue motion over time across a reference line, it is referred to as the M-mode. The M-mode tracing is used for depiction of moving structures such as the cardiac valve but may also be used for evaluation of pleura, pleural fluid and air. The reflected signal from moving echoes may be evaluated using continuous (in CW) or intermittent (in PW) ultrasound beam, with the same being depicted as a graph/waveform (known as spectral Doppler and the graph being known as flow-velocity waveform). If the same signal is converted to a color scale, then it is known as a color Doppler, while if the same signal is superimposed over the gray-scale image, then it may be labelled as duplex Doppler sonography. The term 'Doppler' is used to refer to the basic principle of this type of imaging viz. Doppler shift, whereby the signal towards the insonating probe is seen as 'red' while that going away from probe is seen as 'blue' (and not arterial = red and venous = blue!).

- **Difference between CT thorax and HRCT thorax:** It should be kept in mind that HRCT is a non-contrast non-contiguous scan (mostly of lung but also now of temporal bone and appendix) of three representative regions of lung, which gives an idea of interstitial lung diseases. This technique was developed in times when only conventional (single-slice) CT scans were available, and involves not only acquisition of the image but also post-processing with a special type of software. With the upcoming of spiral/multislice CT scan, the only thing now left is post-processing as the data acquired is otherwise also adequate. Some centres still take it in older algorithm to save radiation exposure to the patient.

- **When should contrast-enhanced CT scan of thorax be done and when is a non-contrast scan sufficient?** With the upcoming of multislice CT scan, injection of intravenous iodinated contrast medium has largely become sparable as most structures can be identified as such. The need for contrast arises in cases of trauma, where contrast extravasation has to be evaluated, or in cases of neoplasias and lymphadenopathy, where enhancement pattern may help in specific diagnosis.

CT scan appearances of common diseases are described in Figures 1.11–1.16.

- **What is multiplanar reconstruction (MPR), maximum intensity projection (MIP), volume rendering (VR) and shaded surface display (SSD)?** These are different kinds of image manipulation/post-processing techniques, which are used to enhance the ability of the reader to view anatomy from different perspectives. This has become possible by the invention of multislice CT scanners, which generate 'isotropic data' (which is uniform in all directions) and thereby can be reconstructed in any anatomical plane (MPR). The CT attenuation values (known as Hounsfield units) of pixels may be separated and pixels of only a specific value may be depicted to generate angiography-like pictures in a technique known as MIP. In VR and SSD the surface features of a 3D structure may be only be depicted.

- **What is a multislice CT (MSCT) and what is a multidetector row CT (MDR-CT)?** The number of detector layers that are arranged opposite to the X-ray tube. We commonly hear people mentioning 16/32/62/128/256 slice CT scan, which refers to the capability of a spiral scanner (one which acquires volume data instead of axial spices) to generate a specific number of slices. It may

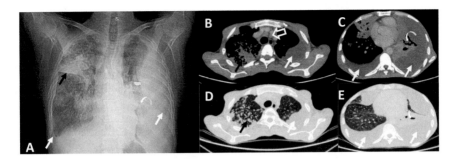

Figure 1.11 (A) Chest radiograph frontal view in supine AP position showing an opacity in right middle zone marked by an inferior straight line (*black arrow*). This indicates towards a consolidation limited by horizontal fissure. Associated patchy, ill-defined, heterogenous and 'soft' (a feature gained by experience only) are seen in whole of right lung. The white arrows mark the dense, homogenous, well-defined opacities are seen in both lungs suggesting pleural effusions. The one of right side shows blunted costo-phrenic angle and is extending upwards along chest wall (due to capillary phenomenon seen in mild to moderate effusion). On the left side an air-bronchogram (*curved arrow*) associated with pleural effusion but no mediastinal shift indicates towards collapse rather than consolidation. These features are also depicted well and confirmed in axial CT scans of chest, mediastinal (B,C) and lung (D,E) windows. An additional finding seen on CT scan is the presence of superior mediastinal lymph nodes between trachea and great vessels (*hollow arrow* in B), an area described as hidden area for chest radiograph.

be remembered that a scanner of 16 rows of detectors may be able to generate 32 slices by way of post-processing of data.

- **BLUE (Bedside Lung Ultrasound in Emergency) protocol (lung assessment for acute respiratory failure):** a 3-minute (time depends on good training under an expert and not just knowledge) protocol done at admission of dyspneic patients, after doing physical examination. A step-wise differential diagnosis of the six main diseases (97% of all cases hence covered) causing acute respiratory failure (pulmonary edema, pulmonary embolism, pneumonia, COPD, asthma, pneumothorax); accuracy = 90.5%.

- **FALLS (Fluid Administration Limited by Lung) protocol (hemodynamic assessment for acute circulatory failure):** echocardiography is the 'heart approach' of assessing circulatory failure due to cardiogenic shock excluding distributive and hypovolemic causes, but is limited by availability of expertise and suitable cardiac windows. BLUE protocol with 'simple heart sonography' (if window available) can also evaluate the presence of the latter two causes/types of shock directly. This may also guide the need for initiating or terminating FALLS. FALLS protocol is a pathophysiology ('Weil's classification of shock')-based 'lung approach' for assessment of the circulatory system as a whole and not 'just cardiac sonography'.

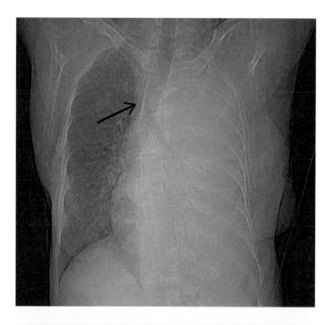

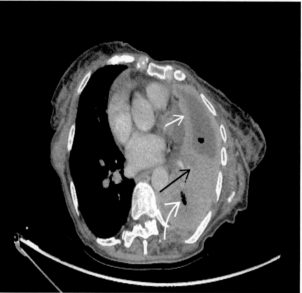

Figure 1.12 Chest X-ray frontal view AP position shows complete opacification of left hemithorax obscuration of left heart border, left hemidiaphragm with mild tracheal shift towards right side (*black arrow*), suggesting complete collapse of left lung with associated massive pleural effusion. On contrast study there is collapse of left lung parenchyma (*white arrow*), with associated moderate pleural effusion (*black arrow*) encapsulated by thickened enhancing pleural lining (*curved white arrow*) having internal foci of air, suggesting empyema. Mild pericardial effusion is also noted.

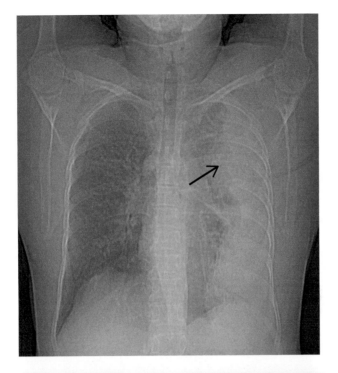

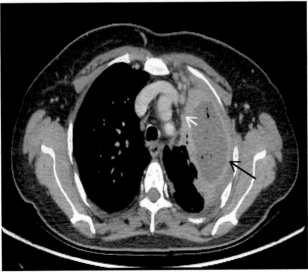

Figure 1.13 Chest X-ray frontal view AP position shows elongated pleural-based concavo-convex opacity (*black arrow*) in left hemithorax, causing volume loss of underlying lung. Axial contrast-enhanced CT thorax image loculated pleural effusion surrounded by thickened enhancing pleura giving 'split pleura sign', s/o empyema (*black arrow*). Few internal air foci are also seen in effusion. There is underlying basal compressive atelectasis (*white arrow*).

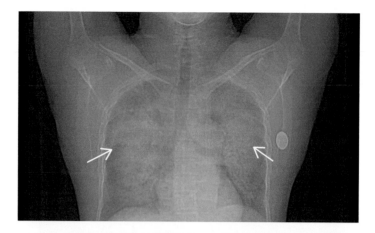

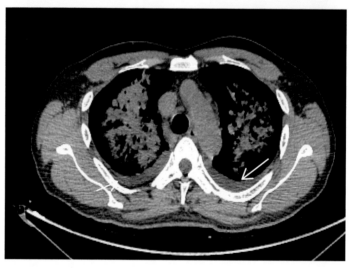

Figure 1.14 Chest X-ray frontal view AP position shows multifocal perihilar and peri-bronchovascular segmental opacities (*white arrow*) in bilateral lung fields with sparing of peripheral subpleural areas (*curved arrow*) giving 'batwing sign', suggesting pulmonary edema. On plain axial CT, multiple confluent segmental and subsegmental patchy consolidations are noted in perihilar location. Bilateral minimal pleural effusion (*white arrow*) is also noted, suggesting pulmonary edema.

DISEASE-BASED REVIEWS

Bronchial asthma

Bronchial asthma is a respiratory disorder characterized by recurrent episodes of wheezing and breathlessness caused by reversible airflow obstruction in association with airway hyper-responsiveness and inflammation triggered by a wide range of stimuli. The intensity and frequency of these episodes are variable.

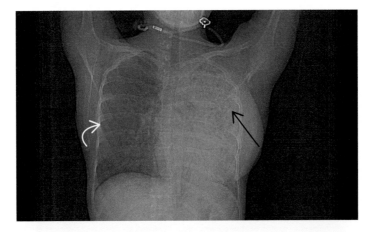

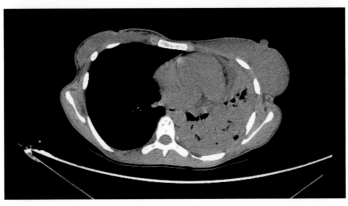

Figure 1.15 Chest radiograph frontal view AP position shows complete opaci-fication of left hemithorax with internal air bronchogram (*black arrow*), no mediastinal shift, left lobar consolidation. Also to note that right-side breast shadow is absent (*curved white arrow*). On plain axial CT, finding of X-ray can be well correlated with clear depiction of consolidation with air bronchogram (*white arrow*).

Q1. Describe the characteristic findings of asthma on chest X-ray.

Answer. Chest X-rays are normal in up to 75% of asthma patients. The following features may be evident on chest X-rays:

- Pulmonary hyperinflation, bronchial wall thickening, parabronchial cuffing and pulmonary edema (in acute severe asthma)
- 'Tram tracks appearance' indicating dilated airways (although more consis-tent with bronchiectasis)
- Horizontally aligned ribs due to continuous outward motion of the upper anterior rib cage during inspiration
- Evidence of pneumothorax, pneumomediastinum and pulmonary edema may be present in acute exacerbations

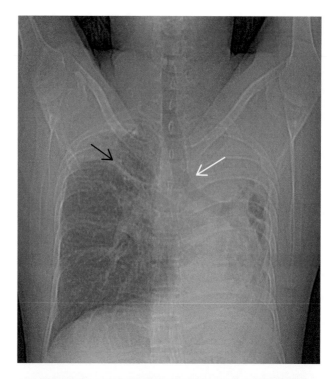

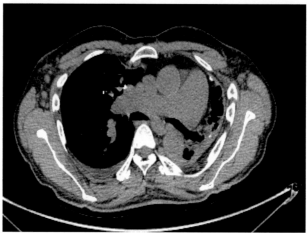

Figure 1.16 Chest X-ray frontal view AP position shows near-complete opacification of left hemithorax with significant volume loss and mediastinal shift to left hemithorax (*white arrow*). Bronchiectatic changes are seen in left middle zone (*black arrow*), suggesting left lung collapse with bronchiectasis. Linear opacity is noted in right upper zone—atelectatic band (*curved arrow*). On plain axial CT, complete collapse of left lung with architectural distortion with fibro-calcific and fibro-bronchiectatic changes. There is volume loss with mediastinal shift on ipsilateral side.

Although chest radiography is not the best imaging modality for asthma, it is a highly effective screening tool during emergency.

Q2. What are the characteristic findings of asthma on computed tomography?
Answer. Although CT imaging has limited usefulness in the diagnosis of bronchial asthma, it can reveal the bronchial wall thickening, narrowing of the bronchial lumen, a reduction in bronchoarterial diameter ratio, small centrilobular opacities, areas of decreased attenuation and vascularity during inspiration and air trapping during expiration.

Q3. What is the usefulness of CT in the diagnosis of asthma-related complications?
Answer. CT scan may be useful in identifying the following features of bronchial asthma:

- *Acute exacerbations*: pneumothorax and pneumomediastinum are the most dreaded complications of acute exacerbation of bronchial asthma. CT chest is very useful for the diagnosis of pneumothorax, especially in asthmatics with an acute decompensation.
- *Complications*: the following complications can occur in asthmatics viz. atelectasis, pneumonia, mucoid impaction, allergic bronchopulmonary aspergillosis (ABPA), bronchocentric granulomatosis, eosinophilic lung disease and Churg-Strauss syndrome. There is also increased incidence of bronchiectasis and emphysema in asthma patients. The following CT findings are useful:

1. ABPA: homogeneous tubular, finger-in-glove or branching endobronchial opacities and bronchiectasis involving mainly the segmental and subsegmental bronchi of the upper lobes, bronchiectasis, centrilobular nodules and mucoid impaction.
2. Chronic eosinophilic pneumonia: characteristic consolidation seen in peripheral lung regions of the middle and upper lung zones bilaterally. Approximately 50% of patients are asthmatics, with women being affected twice as frequently as men.
3. Churg-Strauss syndrome: it is a multisystem disorder characterized by the combination of allergy, peripheral blood eosinophilia and systemic vasculitis. Chest CT findings consist of patchy non-segmental bilateral areas of consolidation or ground-glass opacities with a predominant peripheral distribution. Almost all patients with Churg-Strauss syndrome are asthmatics, and most present with peripheral neuropathy, typically mononeuritis multiplex.
4. Bronchiectasis: bronchiectasis in uncomplicated asthma is typically cylindrical, with broncho-arterial diameter ratio is less than 1.5. CT findings include parallel 'tram tracks' or the 'signet-ring sign', lack of bronchial tapering (including the presence of tubular structures within 1 cm from the pleural surface), bronchial wall thickening in dilated airways, 'tree-in-bud' pattern suggesting inspissated secretions or cysts emanating from the bronchial. Other forms may be varicose or cystic. However, the degree of bronchiectasis does not correlate with the severity of airflow obstruction.

- Airway reversibility: wall-thickness percentage was also inversely correlated with baseline percent predicted forced expiratory volume in one second (FEV1%) and positively correlated with change in FEV1% with bronchodilator challenge.

Chronic Obstructive Pulmonary Disease (COPD)

COPD is an obstructive airway disease characterized by an increase in resistance to airflow due to irreversible partial or complete obstruction, usually occurring in the setting of noxious environmental exposure. It includes emphysema, chronic bronchitis and small airway disease.

- *Emphysema*: irreversible enlargement of the airspaces distal to the terminal bronchiole, accompanied by destruction of their walls without obvious fibrosis (Table 1)
- *Chronic bronchitis*: defined clinically as persistent cough with sputum production for at least 3 months in at least 2 consecutive years, in the absence of any other identifiable cause
- *Small airway disease*: airway disorder characterized by narrowing and reduction of small bronchioles

Q1. What are the characteristic features of COPD on chest X-ray?
Answer. Chest X-ray lacks sensitivity in detecting both airway disease and mild emphysema. However, its low cost, easy accessibility and minimal radiation exposure makes it useful. Both PA and lateral views of chest X-ray are useful. Emphysema and chronic bronchitis are the two basic distinguishable components on chest X-ray.

- Emphysema is characterized by increased radiolucency of the lung fields with or without bullae, flattening of diaphragm, pruning of the peripheral vasculature, increased retrosternal airspace, widening of the intercostal space, narrowed and more vertical cardiac silhouette (Figure 1.8).
- Chronic bronchitis shows only prominent bronchovascular markings.

Q2. What are the characteristic findings of COPD on CT thorax?
Answer.
Chronic bronchitis: bronchial wall thickening, enlarged vessels, repeated inflammation leading to scarring, bronchovascular irregularity and fibrosis
Emphysema: it is seen in four major forms: centriacinar, panacinar, distal acinar and irregular. Of these, only the first two cause clinically significant airflow.
Obstruction: centriacinar emphysema is the most common form, constituting more than 95% of COPD patients.

Table 1.1 Types of Emphysema, Pathophysiology and CT Scan Findings

Type of Emphysema	Involvement	Areas of Involvement	CT Findings
Centriacinar Emphysema	Central or proximal parts of the acini, (respiratory bronchioles), distal alveoli spared	Upper lobes, upper lobes and superior segments of lower lobes	Small well-defined or poorly defined areas of low attenuation surrounded by normal lung. Initially appear as small holes, but become more confluent as the disease progresses.
Panacinar (Panlobular) Emphysema	Uniformly enlarged acini from the level of the respiratory bronchiole to the terminal blind alveoli	Lower lobes and anterior margins of the lung, most severe at the bases	Generalized low attenuation of lung fields suggesting destruction of acini, due to alpha-1 antitrypsin deficiency
Distal Acinar Emphysema	Distal acinus, predominantly involved	Upper and middle lobes, preferably peripheral subpleural lobules adjacent to mediastinal and peripheral pleura with relative sparing of the lung core or central regions	Sub-pleural and peribronchovascular foci of low attenuation separated by intact interlobular septa thickened by associated mild fibrosis
Irregular	Acini are irregularly involved		Irregular areas of hypoattenuation with compensatory over-inflation, invariably associated with scarring

Q3. What other features of COPD are discernible on CT scans apart from emphysema and bronchitis?

Answer. The following features can be associated with COPD:

- Small airway disease: peripheral centrilobular micro-nodular opacities, gas trapping on expiratory CT
- Large airway disease: tracheobronchomalacia, saber sheath appearance, tracheobronchial outpouching/diverticulae
- Interstitial lung disease: patchy ground-glass abnormality, subpleural reticular abnormality
- Pulmonary artery enlargement: suggests pulmonary hypertension, ratio of pulmonary artery to aorta diameter >1, is associated with the risk of COPD exacerbation
- Bronchiectasis

Q4. What are the additional advantages and disadvantages of computed tomography in obstructive airway disorders?

Answer.

Advantages:

- CT is a validated tool for quantification of emphysema and small airway disease in COPD.
- It can estimate the degree of airflow obstruction at pulmonary function testing and the risk of COPD exacerbations by determining bronchial wall thickness and the extent of emphysema.
- It is useful for lung cancer screening, evaluation of pulmonary nodules detected on chest X-ray, assessment of concurrent interstitial lung disease, or planning surgical interventions such as lung transplantation and lung volume reduction surgery (LVRS).
- Helpful in calculating Wall Area Percent (WA%).

Disadvantages: time consuming, radiation exposure

Q5. What is Wall Area Percent (WA%)?

Answer. Wall Area Percent (WA%) is calculated as 100 times the airway wall area divided by the total bronchial cross-sectional area. This has become the standard CT-based measure of airway disease in smokers. Quantitative assessment of the (5th) WA% of more distal airway generations provides stronger correlations to lung function (3rd) than the proximal segmental airway generation), distal measures of WA% provide the strongest correlation to inhaled bronchodilator response in obstructive airway response.

Q6. What are the newer techniques for radiological assessment of airway disorders?

Answer. Magnetic resonance imaging (MRI): use of hyperpolarized gases in MRI offers exciting possibilities for measuring alveolar dimensions. The only major limitation of MRI is the relatively high ratio of air to tissue. The resulting low density of pulmonary hydrogen atoms limits image resolution for the quantitative assessment of structure without the use of intravenous or inhaled contrast-enhancing agents.

Optical Coherence Tomography (OCT): this involves bronchoscopic insertion of a fiber-optic probe into the airways and selectively examining the tracheobronchial tree in detail. However, it may lead to overestimation of the CT measures of airway disease, although it is a sensitive imaging modality to assess disease progression.

FURTHER READING

1. American College of Radiology. *ACR Standard for the Performance of Pediatric and Adult Chest Radiography.* American College of Radiology; 2001.
2. Geitung JT, Skjaerstad LM, Gothlin JH. Clinical utility of chest roentgenograms. *Eur Radiol.* 1999;9:721–3.
3. Rubinowitz AN, Siegel MD, Tocino I. Thoracic imaging in the ICU. *Crit Care Clin.* 2007;23:539–73.
4. Gray P, Sullivan G, Ostryzniuk P, McEwen TAJ, Rigby M, Roberts DE. Value of post procedural chest radiographs in the adult intensive care unit. *Crit Care Med.* 1992;20:1513–18.
5. Expert Round Table on Ultrasound in ICU. International expert statement on training standards for critical care ultrasonography. *Intensive Care Med.* 2011; 37:1077–83.
6. Koenig SJ, Narasimhan M, Mayo PH. Thoracic ultrasonography for the pulmonary specialist. *Chest.* 2011;140:1332–41.
7. Franquet T. Imaging of pneumonia: Trends and algorithms. *Eur Respir J.* 2001;18:196–208.
8. Cameron DC, Borthwick RN, Philp T. The radiographic patterns of acute Mycoplasma pneumonitis. *Clin Radiol.* 1977;28:173–80.
9. Kearney SE, Davies CW, Davies RJ, Gleeson FV. Computed tomography and ultrasound in parapneumonic effusions and empyema. *Clin Radiol.* 2000;55(7):542–7.
10. Sheard S, Rao P, Devaraj A. Imaging of acute respiratory distress syndrome. *Respir Care.* 2012;57(4):607–12.
11. Stein PD, Chenevert TL, Fowler SE, et al. Gadolinium-enhanced magnetic resonance angiography for pulmonary embolism: A multicenter prospective study (PIOPED III). *Ann Intern Med.* 2010;152:434–43.
12. Hill JR, Horner PE, Primack SL. ICU imaging. *Clin Chest Med.* 2008;29:59–76.

2

Cardiovascular system

SANDEEP KAR, KAKALI GHOSH,
PAVAN KUMAR DALLAMPATI AND
ANIRBAN HOM CHOUDHURI

INTRODUCTION

Imaging is one of the essential components of cardiac critical care management. It helps not only in the initial resuscitation, assessment and diagnoses of the condition but also to know the response to treatment. The majority of imaging done bedside in the ICU pertains to cardiac functions. Although initially confined only to the cardiac ICUs, such imaging procedures are currently available in almost all ICUs and are performed routinely.

IMAGING MODALITIES

- Range of cardiac imaging modalities that are available include:
  - Chest radiography
  - Ultrasonography
  - Echocardiography (Echo)
  - Computed tomography (CT)
  - Cardiac magnetic resonance imaging (cardiac MRI)
  - Nuclear scans etc.

Factors affecting the choice of imaging technique

With so many diverse imaging modalities available, the choice of the imaging for a given patient becomes important, which again depends on availability, expertise and cost effectiveness. Whatever imaging modality is used, noninvasiveness and bedside performance are the key benefits of importance to the patient.

DOI: 10.1201/9781003218739-2

Chest radiography

- One of the most common basic imaging techniques done in the ICU due to the availability of portable radiographic machines.
- Helps in identifying the position of central venous catheters, position of the permanent pacemakers, prosthetic valves, intracardiac devices etc. and their complications as well.

- **Central venous catheters**
  - Done for monitoring the central venous pressure as a rough guide to:
    - Volume status
    - Infusion of inotropes, vasopressors
    - Infusion of irritant medications
    - Parenteral nutrition etc.
  - Long-term use in patients receiving chemotherapy, dialysis etc.
  - Complications of CVC insertion include:
    a) Malpositioning of the CVCs is estimated to be up to 5–10%
      - Ideally the tip of the CVC should be present at the junction of superior vena cava and the right atrium, which is visualized in the chest radiograph as just below the anterior first rib.
    b) Misplaced CVC may be present in any of the central systemic veins, such as azygous vein, internal jugular vein (subclavian CVC) etc. or elsewhere
    c) Pneumothorax is the second most common complication, which accounts for up to 6% of all CVC placements (Figure 2.1)
      - A routine chest radiograph is essential for all successful or unsuccessful placements of CVC. So, if a patient is scheduled for routine chest radiography, it should be taken only after attempting for CVC.
      - A lateral radiograph is obtained in patients for confirmation of a misplaced tip in the azygous vein or in upright position for finding a very small pneumothorax.
    d) Vascular injury
      - May present as new-onset pleural collection.
      - May be due to:
        - Hemothorax
        - Misdirection of the catheter
        - Mediastinal hematoma as mediastinal widening
        - Extrapleural hematoma (apical cap) etc.
      - Contrast injection through the central venous catheter is required sometimes to document the vascular injury and misplacement
    e) Knotting, coiling, kinking, thrombosis causes further complications
    f) Fragmentation because of compression between clavicle and first rib called pinch-off syndrome, which can also be detected by chest radiography

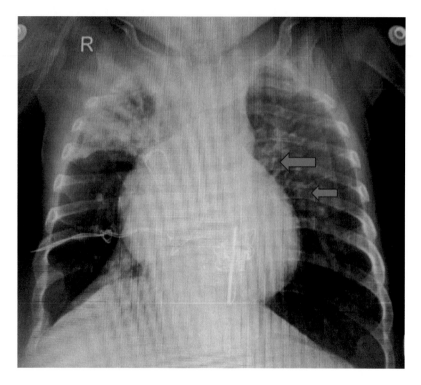

Figure 2.1 Pneumothorax (*blue arrow* showing lung margin).

- **Heart silhouette (Figure 2.2)**
  - Right heart border: The right heart is identified, and it is followed from the diaphragm. From diaphragm to the hilum, the right heart border is formed by the right atrium. From hilum upwards, it is formed by the superior vena cava.
  - Left heart border: From the diaphragm up to the hilum, left heart border is formed by the left ventricle. At the lower level of left hilum, the left border is concave and is formed by the left atrial appendage. In patients with left atrial enlargement, there is loss of this concavity and hence the left heart border is either straightened or convexity ensues. At the hilum, the border is formed by the left pulmonary artery and above it by the aortic knuckle.
  - To differentiate the mitral and aortic valves, a line is drawn from the right cardiophrenic angle to the left atrial appendage. The valve above this line would be the aortic and below would be the mitral.
  - Lateral films are useful in identifying the posterior border of the heart, which is formed by the left ventricle and the anterior border formed by the right ventricle.

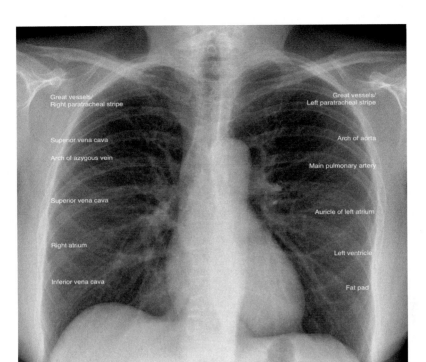

Figure 2.2 Heart silhouette.

- To differentiate the mitral and aortic valves in lateral films, a line is drawn from apex of the heart to the hilum or carina, valve above this line will be aortic and below will be mitral.

- **Pulmonary embolus**
  - An area in lung which is blacker than the other side at the same level depicting an area of reduced perfusion to that area of lung due to a clot in the artery supplying that area, also called "Westermark's sign" (Figure 2.3).

- **Hilar enlargement**
  - Unilateral hilar dilatation may be due to:
    - Pulmonary artery aneurysm
    - Post-stenotic dilatation of the pulmonary artery
    - Other mediastinal causes
  - Bilateral hilar enlargement may be due to:
    - Primary pulmonary hypertension where both hila look convex and peripheral pruning in the lung fields (reduction in peripheral vascularity with edges with the lung field edges are lighter and central fields whiter than usual).

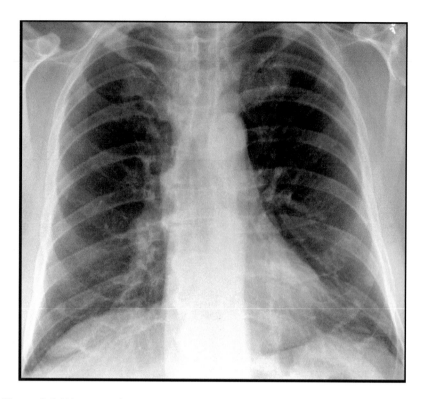

Figure 2.3 Westermark's sign.

SPECIFIC CARDIAC LESIONS ON CXR

- *Atrial septal defect*
  - Heart enlargement (determined by the cardiothoracic ratio by measuring the width of the thorax and the width of the heart if it is more than half the diameter of thorax) along with pulmonary hypertension.
  - The apex will be rounded due to right ventricular enlargement.
  - Might be lifted off from the diaphragm, and the right heart border is fuller than usual due to right atrial enlargement.
  - The position of heart may be shifted to left so that the right edge of the vertebral column is seen.
  - Smaller aortic knuckle due to the diversion of blood to right atrium.
  - Mitral stenosis (Figure 2.4): loss of concavity just below the left hilum due to the left atrial enlargement often straightening the left heart border or even makes it convex.
  - "The double right heart border" due to left atrial enlargement.
  - Elevation of left main bronchus due to left atrial enlargement causes the angle between the carina and the left bronchus to be more than 90°.

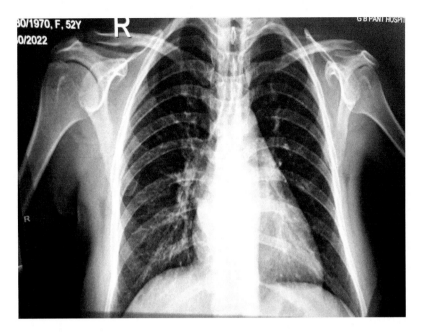

Figure 2.4 CXR showing straightening of left heart border.

Other classic chest radiography signs of congenital cardiac lesions include:

- "Egg on string sign" in transposition of great arteries.
- "Snowman's sign" in total anomalous pulmonary venous return.
- "Scimitar sign" in partial anomalous venous return.
- "Gooseneck sign" in endocardial cushion defects.
- "Boot-shaped heart" in tetralogy of Fallot.
- "Figure of three and reverse figure of three" in coarctation of aorta.
- "Box-shaped heart" in Epstein anomaly.
- Interpretation of heart size and shape of the mediastinum may not be accurate in an AP view as both are distorted and lying position of the patient makes it more erroneous to interpret.
- The disadvantages of chest radiography are that they have low sensitivity, exposure to radiation, fetal exposure is not desirable hence a relative contraindication in pregnancy.

Ultrasonography

- Bedside ultrasonography gives rapid and real-time answers about patients.
- Cardiac ultrasonography is a part of point-of-care ultrasonography (POCUS). It is successful in critical care units because it is:

- Relatively inexpensive
- Radiation free
- Painless
- Has fewer logistical issues compared to that of portable radiography
- Ease of learning by non-radiologists especially intensivists which brought immediacy, repeatability and integration

- Disadvantages are quality images rely on skill and persistence of the sonographer.
- Used extensively pertaining to cardiac invasive procedures in ICU such as guiding the insertion of central venous catheters, guiding pericardial paracentesis.
- The abdominal ultrasonography is used for the assessment of vascular structures such as abdominal aorta aneurysms or dissections, hemodynamic assessment.

Abdominal aorta: Abdominal Aortic Aneurysm (AAA)

- If ruptured, it will be a catastrophic event.
- Identification of AAA is very crucial in cases of persistent hypotension, abdominal pain and unilateral hydronephrosis; an ultrasound examination is specific and sensitive in detecting AAA.
- The normal aorta size is 3 cm, and the risk of rupture would be low if it is less than 4 cm. The risk increases rapidly if the diameter is more than 5.5 cm.
  - Volume status and inferior vena cava (IVC) collapsibility:
    - IVC is very sensitive to fluid changes as it is collapsible and the diameter changes with respiratory changes of intrathoracic pressures.
    - IVC diameters are measured and IVC collapsibility index in spontaneously breathing, but IVC distensibility index is calculated in mechanically ventilated patients.
    - IVC distensibility index in a ventilated patient are calculated as clinical parameter to assess the fluid status of the patient.
    - With the probe in the subxiphoid region, IVC is identified where it joins the right atrium. It is traced back up to a point beyond where the hepatic veins drain into IVC. Here M-mode is applied and the minimum IVC diameter on inspiration and the maximum diameter of IVC on expiration are measured in spontaneously breathing patient.
    - The reverse applies in mechanically ventilated patient.

$$\text{IVC collapsibility index} = \text{Max IVC diameter on expiration} - \frac{\text{Min IVC diameter on insp}}{\text{Max IVC diameter on exp}}$$

$$\text{IVC distensibility index} = \frac{\text{Max IVC diameter on inspiration} - \text{Min IVC diameter on exp}}{\text{Min IVC diameter on exp}}$$

  - An IVC collapsibility index of more than 50% is associated with severe dehydration and need for fluid therapy.

Echocardiography

- Considered as the "extension of examining hand" as it provides real-time images in finding quick answers in critical care setup.
- Echocardiography is used in ICU for the assessment of:
  - Hemodynamics
  - Fluid responsiveness
  - Procedural guidance
  - Diagnosis of shock
  - In cardiac arrest
  - In extracorporeal life support
  - In ventricular assist devices etc.

- Echocardiography can be viewed as an extension of the routine ultrasonography but limited to heart and its major vessels.
- Focused echocardiography is done at the bedside often serially in rapid succession by the critical care physician and is called focused critical care echocardiography (FCCE).
- Used to rapidly answer specific practical, straightforward clinical questions such as fluid responsiveness, pericardial effusion, inotropic responsiveness etc., what is called goal-directed echocardiography.
- Transesophageal echocardiography is only used as an adjunct to echocardiography despite its superior image quality, because of the:
  - Invasive nature of insertion
  - Maintenance of the equipment
  - Prolonged learning curve
  - To be inserted only in mechanically ventilated patients or in deep sedation

BASIC TRANSTHORACIC ECHOCARDIOGRAPHY VIEWS

Some of the basic views every critical care physician should know are as follows:

- *Parasternal long axis view (PLAX)* (Figure 2.5): place the probe marker towards right shoulder in the 2nd or 3rd intercostal space near the left sternal border. In this view, the left atrium, mitral valve, left ventricle, the interventricular septum, right ventricle, aortic valve, and the ascending aorta are seen in long axis.
- *Short axis view* (Figures 2.6, 2.7): from PLAX if the probe is rotated 90° with the pointer towards the left shoulder, the short axis views are obtained. To get the aortic short axis view, the probe is slightly tilted towards the head. Here we can see the aorta in the short axis (Mercedes Benz sign), right atrium, tricuspid valve, right ventricle, right ventricle outflow tract (RVOT), the pulmonary artery and part of LA. Similarly, if the probe is tilted towards the apex, LV short axis is viewed at different levels, namely valvular level, papillary level and apical level.
- *Four-chamber view* (Figure 2.8): place the probe to the lateral of the apex with the marker towards the left shoulder. In this view the right atrium, tricuspid valve, right ventricle, interventricular septum, left atrium, mitral valve and left

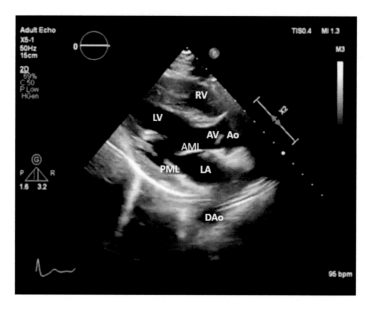

Figure 2.5 Parasternal long axis view (PLAX) (LV: left ventricle, RV: right ventricle, AML: anterior mitral leaflet, Ao: aortic outlet, Dao: descending aorta, PML: post-mitral leaflet, LA: left atrium, RA: right atrium).

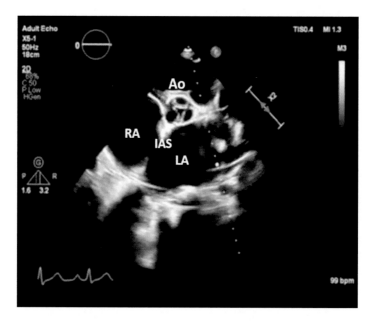

Figure 2.6 Parasternal short axis view at aortic valve level (Ao: aortic outlet, RA: right atrium, IAS: interatrial septum, LA: left atrium).

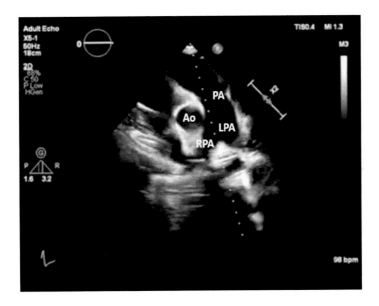

Figure 2.7 Parasternal short axis view (Ao: aortic outlet, PA: pulmonary artery, RPA: right pulmonary artery, LPA: left pulmonary artery).

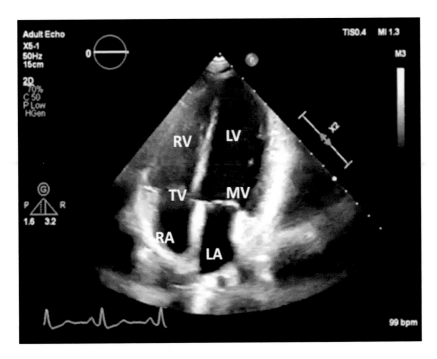

Figure 2.8 Apical four-chambered view (RV: right ventricle, LV: left ventricle, RA: right atrium, LA: left atrium, TV: tricuspid valve, MV: mitral valve).

ventricle will be seen. In the same view if we tilt the probe ventrally, the LVOT and the aorta starts opening, and this view is called five-chamber view.

- *Subcostal view*: place the probe below the xiphoid notch slightly to the right and the pointer towards the left hip. Gentle pressure must be used so that the ultrasound beam passes beneath the sternum and ribs to view the heart.

HEMODYNAMIC EVALUATION BY ECHOCARDIOGRAPHY

Defining the hemodynamic variations that occur commonly in critically ill patients, the response to the interventions and targeted management thereof is the primary role of echocardiography in critical care.

Measuring the right heart pressures can be achieved either by catheterization, which is an invasive procedure, or by simple non-invasive echocardiography.

- *Fluid responsiveness*
  - Defined as an increase in stroke volume by 10–15% after volume expansion by intravascular fluid administration.
  - Intravascular fluid administration is a double-edged sword in that it treats the hypovolemia, but excess fluid may cause respiratory and renal failure in an already compromised system. Hence fluid management is to be dealt with utmost care in critical care patients.
  - The goal in assessing fluid responsiveness is to differentiate patients whose stroke volume increases with fluid challenge and whose might not benefit from fluid administration.

- *Central venous pressure*
  - Determined by IVC collapsibility index or IVC distensibility index.
  - Superior vena caval distensibility of 36% is also shown be a predictor of fluid responsiveness.

- *Pulmonary artery pressure*
  - In the presence of pulmonary hypertension, it is expected that there would be tricuspid regurgitation (TR) in correlation with the degree of pulmonary hypertension.
  - Using the modified Bernoulli's equation, the measurement of right ventricular systolic pressure (RVSP) is estimated from TR peak jet velocity given that there is absence of pulmonary stenosis.
  - Another method of measuring pulmonary artery pressure in the absence of tricuspid regurgitation is by using pulmonary velocity acceleration time.
  - It is achieved by looking at the pulse wave (PW) Doppler signal of the pulmonary blood flow at the pulmonary valve level. Its maximum velocity is in the range of 0.8–1.2 m/sec.
  - The time interval between the onset of the flow to the peak is called pulmonary velocity acceleration time (PVAT). When the pulmonary pressure and the pulmonary vascular resistance are high, there will be an early peak.

- The normal PVST is > 130 millisec signifies normal pulmonary artery pressure (PAP), 100–130 millisec: borderline PAP, 80–100 millisec: mildly elevated PAP and < 80 millisec signifies severe PAP.
- PVAT measurement is valid when the heart rate is between 60–100, there is no increased right ventricular flow as in atrial septal defect and absence of severe pulmonary regurgitation.

- *Diagnosis and management of shock*
  - Shock is a condition where tissue hypoperfusion may lead to organ damage.
  - There are many types of shock where management changes from one condition to another.
  - In critical care with a rapidly deteriorating patient, the etiology might be undifferentiated shock, or it may be multifactorial. The prompt diagnosis and its treatment will be the key in saving such patients.
  - Most common causes are:
    - Left ventricular failure (acute valvular dysfunction, intracardiac mass, hypertrophic obstructive cardiomyopathy, outflow tract obstruction etc.)
    - Acute cor pulmonale
    - Pericardial tamponade
    - Hypovolemic shock
    - Septic shock

- *Left ventricular failure*
  - One of the etiologies of shock
  - May be the result of:
    - Ischemic heart disease
    - Non-ischemic cardiomyopathy
    - Global hypoxemia
    - Metabolic derangements
    - Toxic derangements etc.
  - Estimation of ejection fraction (EF) is the most common assessment of global function of left ventricle by several methods such as:
    - Two-dimensional planimetry (modified Simpson method)
    - M-mode in SAX view (Teichholz formula)
    - Fractional shortening
    - Fractional area contraction
    - Mitral annulus post-systolic excursion (MAPSE)
    - dP/dT
    - Eyeballing
  - The principle behind measuring the ejection fraction is ejected volume is dependent on left ventricle end diastolic volume (LVEDV) and the normal value is more than 55%.

$$LVEF = \frac{LV \text{ end diastolic volume } (LVEDV) - LV \text{ end systolic volume } (LVESV)}{LV \text{ end diastolic volume } (LVEDV)}$$

Two-dimensional method

The left ventricular end diastolic and systolic volumes are calculated by tracing the left ventricular endocardium in both end diastole and end systole. By using the prior formula, the ejection fraction is calculated.

Motion mode or M-mode

M-mode is the time motion display of the ultrasound wave along the ultrasound line, which provides a mono-dimensional view of the heart where all the reflectors in the line are displayed along the time axis.

Fractional Shortening (FS)

$$FS = \frac{\text{LV end diastolic diameter } (LVEDD) - \text{LV end systolic diameter } (LVESD)}{LVEDD} \times 100$$

- Normal FS = 25–40%
- Fractional area contraction (FAC)
- By pacing the M-mode in the LV SAX

$$FAC = \frac{\text{LV end diastolic area } (LVEDA) - \text{LV end systolic area } (LVESA)}{LVEDA} \times 100$$

- Normal FAC is 35–45%

Mitral Annular Post-systolic Excursion (MAPSE)

Measuring the systolic movement of the mitral annular ring is one of the quickest methods to estimate the LVEF. In the apical four-chamber view, the M-mode cursor is placed on the lateral mitral annulus, and the excursion of the mitral valve during systole and diastole are measured. The normal MAPSE > 10 mm correlates with EF > 55%.

- *Two-dimensional planimetry (modified Simpsons method)*
  - Right heart failure due to increased resistance to the pulmonary blood flow is cor pulmonale.
  - Critical care physicians deal with acute cor pulmonale often as a complication of pulmonary embolism and acute respiratory distress syndrome.
  - It can be documented in echocardiography by:
    - RV to LV end diastolic ratio > 1
    - RV FAC < 35%
    - Tricuspid annular plane systolic exertion (TAPSE) < 16mm
    - Eccentricity index >1 (D-shaped interventricular septum)
    - Right ventricular systolic pressure measured as tricuspid regurgitation > 35 mm Hg etc.
  - TAPSE and eccentricity index need a special mention.
    - TAPSE: measured by placing the M-mode on the lateral tricuspid annulus towards the apex in a four-chamber view and measuring the

distance between the end diastole to the end systole. Even though the RVOT, IVS is not included in the measurement, which contribute significantly to the RV function, it gives a fair idea about the RV function.

– Eccentricity index: to identify the RV volume overload to pressure load as there will be abnormal motion of inter-ventricular septum in both conditions, eccentricity index is measured. Two minor axes are taken in the SAX view of the LV, one axis parallel to the IVS and the other perpendicular to it. The ratio of parallel axis to the perpendicular axis measured in both end systole and end diastole gives us the eccentricity ratio. In normal subjects, the ratio at both end systole and diastole will be 1.0 as LV in SAX will be circular in the absence of RV disease (abnormal IVS). In RV volume overload, the index at end systole will be 1.0 but will be increased in end diastole. In patients with RV pressure overload, the eccentricity index will be more than 1.0 in both end systole and end diastole.

- *Pulmonary embolism (PE)* (Figure 2.9)
  - PE is best diagnosed by CT, ventilation-perfusion scans.
  - Relative contra indication in cases of patient's instability, poor renal parameters and significant pulmonary disease makes echocardiography an alternative.
  - Two important signs which are characteristic of RV dysfunction in patients of PE need special mention:

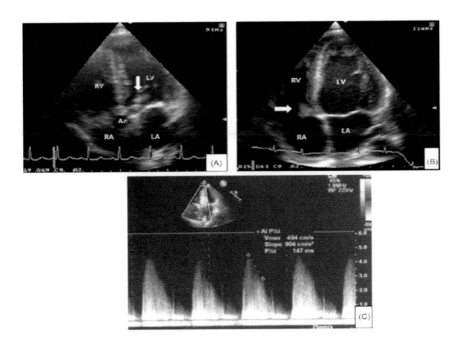

Figure 2.9 (A) arrow showing thrombus in LV, (B) arrow showing thrombus between RA and RV (C).

- McConnell's sign refers to free ventricular hypokinesis with apical sparing.
- 60–60 sign refers to right ventricular acceleration time ≤ 60 millisec in conjunction with tricuspid regurgitation with pressure gradient ≤ 60 mm of Hg.

- *Pericardial tamponade*
  - Rare cause of undifferentiated shock, which needs prompt diagnosis and drainage.
  - The characteristic echocardiographic findings in tamponade are:
    - Pericardial effusion
    - Plethoric IVC
    - RA systolic collapse
    - RV diastolic collapse
    - Septal bounce
    - 60% inspiratory decrease in tricuspid peak E wave velocity
    - 30% decrease in inspiratory mitral peak E wave velocity

- *Hypovolemic shock*
  - In severe hypovolemia, echocardiographic features are:
    - Small and collapsible IVC
    - Supranormal LVEF
    - Kissing walls of LV (complete collapse of LV during systole in SAX)
    - Small LV end diastolic area
    - Dynamic interventricular outflow obstruction

- *Septic shock*
  - Causes may be:
    - LV strain
    - LV systolic dysfunction
    - LV diastolic dysfunction
    - RV systolic dysfunction
    - RV diastolic dysfunction

- *Cardiac arrest*
  - Echocardiography is used both as a diagnostic and prognostic tool in cardiac arrest and IIb recommendation in ACLS protocol.
  - Echocardiography is used to diagnose the reversible causes of cardiac arrest.
  - Focused echocardiographic evaluation during life support (FEEL protocol) is a structured approach in cardiac arrest scenarios in which subcostal view is obtained during a pulse check without prolonging breaks between chest compression, which are associated with improved outcome.

Computed tomography

- The practice of medicine has changed tremendously with the introduction of computed tomography in modern medicine.

- Very short acquisition times help the clinician to use CT for evaluation of vascular disorders such as aortic dissection, pulmonary embolism etc.
- Despite being an excellent diagnostic tool, mobilizing the sick patient in ICU poses a significant risk.
- The invention of portable CT machines (CT scan on wheels) has unveiled a new era of CT in ICU, which is eliminating the logistic issues and getting closer to the critical care patients' needs.
- CT scan can be viewed as a higher version of radiography with higher detail, 360-degree view.

- *Two-dimensional planimetry (modified Simpsons method)* (Figure 2.10)
  - The hallmarks of cardiac failure would be similar to those of radiography.
  - Provides a higher detail such as cardiac chamber dilatation, pulmonary vascular engorgement, pleural effusion, interstitial pulmonary edema.
  - Specific uses of CT in relation to heart would be evaluation of:
    - Ischemic heart disease
    - Calcium deposition in the coronary arteries, aorta
    - Pericardial effusion
    - Pulmonary vasculature
    - Heart valves
    - Heart function
  - One of the prerequisites for cardiac CT is low heart rate without arrythmias, or otherwise will be having motion artifacts.
  - Breath holding for 15–20 seconds is needed for a better-quality image.

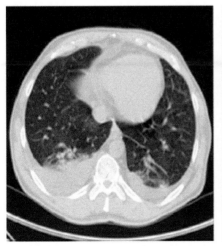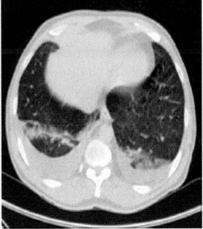

Figure 2.10 Axial CT of the lower thorax with lung window settings shows mild bilateral pleural effusion with passive atelectasis of underlying lungs.

Coronary angiography

- Newest in the development of cardiac CT.
- 64-channel angiography gives greater craniocaudal coverage per rotation and hence a shorter breath hold is required, as well as a small volume of contrast injection, less heart variability.
- 64-slice CT has a better special and temporal resolution and hence superior performance. There are many limitations in cardiac CT.
- "Blooming effect" refers to overestimation of volume set representing calcium in patients with extensive coronary plaque calcifications. So symptomatic patients with severe calcium scores are subjected to invasive coronary angiogram directly. Detection of restenosis in stents of the size of 3 mm is limited.
- The greatest applicability of coronary CT is in differentiating acute chest pain from coronary (obstructive coronary artery disease) and non-coronary (aortic dissection, pulmonary embolism) etiology in emergency situations.
- As the caliber of the coronary artery bypass grafts is larger than the naive coronary vessels and are prone to less motion artifact, their evaluation by coronary CT has gained much importance in recent times.
- Usage of metallic clips may cause artifacts, and the distal anastomoses are less clearly viewed.
- In addition to coronary anomalies, coronary artery aneurysm, arterio-venous fistula, myocardial bridges can be easily reconstructed in three-dimensional CT.
- Cardiac masses: the location, extent of spread, vascularity, anatomic relation to other cardiac and non-cardiac structures can be well documented in cardiac CT.
- The left atrial appendage thrombi can also be detected with high sensitivity but with low specificity.
- Pericardial thickness and tissue characteristics can be well determined by the cardiac CT.

Myocardial Perfusion Scintigraphy (MPS)

- MPS looks at the blood flow changes with stress.
- It depends on the principle that on physical stress, the oxygen demand increases, which leads to coronary vasodilatation and increase in the blood flow in the healthy arteries.
- In stenosed arteries, despite increase in demand, there will be no increase in blood flow, which leads to myocardial ischemia and symptoms thereof.
- In patients who cannot do exercise, pharmacological stress testing can be done by giving Dobutamine or Dypyridamole or Adenosine.
- Newer imaging techniques such as sequential CT, single photon emission computed tomography (SPECT) and positron emission tomography (PET) have been developed, which provide better blood flow information in less time.
- Also provides better information regarding left ventricular perfusion, volumes, ejection fraction and diastolic function.

- We can plan the position of various cardiac devices due to information by MPS on perfusion, ventricular systolic and diastolic function with phase and movement asynchrony combining with CT anatomy information from hybrid images.
- With the newer agents available such as ^{123}I-labelled meta-iodobenzyl guanidine (MIBG), which is a noradrenaline analogue that is stored in myocardial presynaptic adrenergic nerve terminal.
- By measuring uptake and washout of MIBG, sympathetic innervation of myocardium can be assessed.
- This is particularly useful in assessing the symptoms and left ventricular ejection fraction in risk stratification and prognostication of patients with cardiac failure.

Ischemic memory imaging

- In normal physiological conditions, fatty acids are the major substrate for the myocardium. During ischemia there will be preferential shift of metabolism from fatty acids to the glucose. This shift may persist for 12 hours after ischemia has subsided.
- ^{123}I-labelled 15–(p-iodophenyl)-3R, S-methylpentadecanoic acid (BMIPP) is an iodinated fatty acid with high normal uptake and delayed retention by myocardium.
- Hence, BMIPP is used to image the past ischemic event! Combining the [99]Tc[m] perfusion scan with ^{123}I fatty acid scan can eliminate the need for stress tests in patients with suspected acute coronary syndrome.

MRI

- Cardiac MRI is a highly accurate, non-ionizing method for assessing cardiac function and morphology.
- Its ability to characterize tissue is useful to define the morphological nature of scar, inflammation and necrosis, and hence it is well established for the diagnosis and follow-up of cardiomyopathies and myocarditis.
- It is used in conjunction with echocardiography for the diagnosis and follow-up of congenital cardiac diseases.
- Cardiac MRI is superior to SPECT in terms of assessment of myocardial perfusion.
- MRI is the most accurate modality of assessing the myocardial infarction both in acute and chronic phases.
- Can differentiate between the myocardial hibernation and viability.
- For non-invasive imaging of the coronary arteries, though CT is superior to the MRI, because of its ionizing hazard, MRI is accepted as an alternative.
- Disadvantages of MRI include:
  - Breath holding is required
  - Difficulty getting in and out of the scanner in patients with multiple problems

- Heating up tip of the implantable cardiac devices
- Poor image quality in arrythmias
- Renal toxicity with gadolinium-based late enhancement scans

FURTHER READING

1. Tsotsolis N, Tsirgogianni K, Kioumis I, et al. Pneumothorax as a complication of central venous catheter insertion. *Ann Transl Med.* 2015;3(3):40.
2. Oren-Grinberg A, Talmor D, Brown SM. Focused critical care echocardiography. *Crit Care Med.* 2013;41(11):2618–26.
3. Miller A, Mandeville J. Predicting and measuring fluid responsiveness with echocardiography. *Echo Res Pract.* 2016;3(2):G1–G12.
4. Lang RM, Bierig M, Devereux RB, Flachskampf FA, Foster E, Pellikka PA, Picard MH, Roman MJ, Seward J, Shanewise J, Solomon S, Spencer KT, St. John Sutton M, Stewart W. Recommendations for chamber quantification. *Eur J Echocardiogr.* 2006;7(2):79–108.
5. Chengode S. Left ventricular global systolic function assessment by echocardiography. *Ann Card Anaesth.* 2016;19(Suppl):S26–S34.
6. Bergenzaun L, Öhlin H, Gudmundsson P, et al. Mitral annular plane systolic excursion (MAPSE) in shock: A valuable echocardiographic parameter in intensive care patients. *Cardiovasc Ultrasound.* 2013;11:16.
7. Shah BR, Velamakanni SM, Patel A, Khadkikar G, Patel TM, Shah SC. Analysis of the 60/60 sign and other right ventricular parameters by 2D transthoracic echocardiography as adjuncts to diagnosis of acute pulmonary embolism. *Cureus.* 2021;13(3):e13800.
8. Pérez-Casares A, Cesar S, Brunet-Garcia L, Sanchez-de-Toledo J. Echocardiographic evaluation of pericardial effusion and cardiac tamponade. *Front Pediatr.* 2017;5:79.
9. Flower L, Olusanya O, Madhivathanan PR. The use of critical care echocardiography in peri-arrest and cardiac arrest scenarios: Pros, cons and what the future holds. *J Intensive Care Soc.* 2021;22(3):230–40.

3

Nervous system

ISHAN KUMAR, ASHISH VERMA
AND BHUVNA AHUJA

NEUROIMAGING MODALITIES

CT and MRI are the primary neuroimaging modalities, with an adjunctive role of Doppler ultrasound and digital subtraction angiography (DSA) in some patients.

Computed tomography

Relies on the differential attenuation of X-ray by body tissues of differing density.
- *Advantage*: it is fast and easily available

- *Non-contrast CT*: reveals bony abnormalities, acute hemorrhage, cerebral edema, hydrocephalus, mass effect, acute infarct

- *Contrast-enhanced CT*: requires administration of iodinated contrast media through intravenous route. It is useful for neoplastic, infectious and vascular abnormalities of the brain and spinal cord
  - For CECT head, 80 mL contrast (1.5 mL/sec) is administered intravenously and the scan is obtained approximately 2 min after injection

- *CT angiography: arterial evaluation*
  - 80 mL contrast (4 mL/sec) is administered and scan is performed in arterial phase using bolus chasing technique.
  - Usually both brain and carotid angiography is performed.

- *CT venography: evaluation of veins*
  - 80 mL contrast (4 mL/sec) is given and scan is performed 45 seconds after giving contrast.

DOI: 10.1201/9781003218739-3

- *CT perfusion*: is similarly undertaken to look for ischemic penumbra
  - 40 mL contrast (6 mL/sec).
- *In CT head*, the image is obtained in the axial plane and coronal and sagittal reconstruction is done.
- *Volume-rendered images*: three-dimensional representation of data.
- *Maximum intensity projection*: the highest density values from the CT data are used to create angiographic images.

- Patients undergoing CT with IV contrast require a serum creatinine in acceptable range with the exception of in emergent situations. Risk of contrast-induced nephropathy should always be evaluated by calculating eGFR using MDRD formula
  - EGFR >45 mL/min/1.73 m^2: full-dose contrast
  - EGFR: 30–45 mL/min/1.73 m^2: full-dose contrast with hydration
  - EGFR <30 mL/min/1.73 m^2: avoid contrast. If needed absolutely, give prophylactic hydration
  - Patients on metformin, if EGFR <30 mL/min/1.73 m^2, discontinue metformin at the time of scan and restart after 48 hours of giving contrast
  - Patients on routine dialysis, correlation of contrast administration with timing of hemodialysis is not necessary
  - Prefer using Visipaque in patients with renal dysfunction

- The estimated radiation dose for a CT head is 2 mGy (<50 mGy radiation dose in pregnant women does not carry significant risk of malignancy, miscarriage, major fetal malformation).

Magnetic resonance imaging

- Consists of a large, powerful magnet in which the patient lies. It uses non-ionizing radiation to create useful diagnostic images.
- It uses the magnetic properties of hydrogen nucleus (proton) in water and fat. When the body is placed in a strong magnetic field (B^0 e.g. 1.5 Tesla or 3 Tesla), the protons all line up in the direction of the MR scanner. When additional energy (radiofrequency pulse) is added to the magnetic field 90^0 to the B$_0$, the magnetic vector is deflected. When the radiofrequency source is switched off, the magnetic vector returns to its resting state, and this causes a signal (also a radio wave) to be emitted. This signal is used to create the MR images. Different tissues relax at different rates, leading to image contrast.
- There are few absolute contraindications of MRI, such as presence of a mobile internal metallic foreign body (such as bullet fragment in abdomen or ocular foreign body, cochlear implant, subcutaneous insulin pump), most cardiac pacemakers. All other devices are MR safe, including bony implants, cardiac valves, aneurysm coils/clips, stents. All metallic objects or electronic devices of the patients should be preferably removed prior to entering MRI department.
- On MRI, various pulse sequences have been designed. Four basic MR sequences used in almost all patients are T1, T2, fluid-attenuated inversion recovery (FLAIR) and diffusion-weighted imaging (DWI). T1-weighted images are good for showing anatomical details and hemorrhage and comparison with

post-contrast T1 images. T2 and FLAIR are useful in depicting edema and other pathological processes. DWI can identify cytotoxic edema (infarct, abscess, epidermoid). SWI or GRE sequences are very useful if hemorrhage or calcification is suspected.

- Contrast-enhanced MRI is performed using administration of gadolinium-based contrast media. Gadolinium-based MRI contrast agent is administered intravenously in approximately 0.2 mL/kg (0.1 mmoles/kg) at a rate of 10 mL per 15 seconds. Contrast should be avoided in patients with eGFR < 30 mL/min/1.73 m^2 because of the risk of nephrogenic systemic fibrosis (scleroderma-like skin manifestations). If absolutely needed, prefer using macro-cyclic contrast (Dotarem) or less preferably Multihance. MRI examination should be scheduled just ahead of hemodialysis session.
- MR angiography and MR venography can be done without giving contrast and is a better alternative than CT angiography for patients with renal disease.

PRINCIPLES OF INTERPRETATION OF HEAD CT (TABLE 3.1)

- On CT, the density or brightness of a tissue is represented using Hounsfield unit (HU).
- Water has a HU value of zero. Bone has a HU value of +1000 and air has a value of –1000 HU.
- Contrast CT images should be viewed with non-contrast to identify true enhancement (increase in CT attenuation by more than 20 HU) from non-enhancing hyperattenuating tissue.
- "Windowing" is a process to highlight the tissue of interest (Figure 3.1).
  - Brain window: brain parenchyma, ventricles
  - Bone window: used for bones and air-filled structures such as sinuses, pneumocephalus
  - Soft tissue window: orbits

Table 3.1 Basics of CT Appearances of Various CNS Structures

Isodense	White matter	+25 HU
	Gray matter	+40 HU
	Muscle, soft tissue	+20 to 40 HU
	Subacute bleed	
Hyperdense/hyperattenuating	Intracranial hemorrhage	60 to 100
	Punctate calcifications	30 to 500
	Iodinated CT contrast	100 to 600
	Bone, calcium, metal	1000 or more
Hypodense	CSF, cyst, old bleeds	+15
Hypoattenuating	Fat	–30 to –70
	Air	– 1000

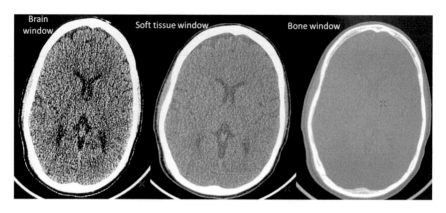

Figure 3.1 CT images of same patient in different CT windows (i.e. brain window, soft tissue window and bone window respectively).

PRINCIPLES OF INTERPRETATION OF MRI OF BRAIN

How are MRI sequences identified and what are the common indications of each sequence (see Figures 3.2 and 3.3)? Table 3.2 summarizes the common sequences and their indications.

Characteristics of tissues under MRI sequencing

How are various tissues characterized using different MRI sequences?

- Tissue brighter than brain parenchyma on any sequence is called hyperintense and darker tissue is called hypointense.
- Lesions that are bright on DWI and dark on ADC are referred to as exhibit diffusion restriction. Acute infarct, hemorrhage, abscess, epidermoid and highly cellular tumors show diffusion restriction.
- Areas that are extremely dark on GRE or SWI are identified as area of "blooming" and represent hemorrhage/calcification.
- Lesions or areas which show increased brightness on post-contrast images compared to T1 sequence are said to show post-contrast enhancement.
- Edema: edema appears hyperintense on T2/FLAIR and hypointense on T1.
- Hemorrhage: show different signal depending on age of hemorrhage. In acute/early subacute phase, these are dark on T2 and bright to isointense on T1, show restriction. Susceptibility weighted images (SWI) are best to detect hemorrhage where they show blooming.
- Fat: appears bright on both T1/T2 sequence. To differentiate edema from fat from pathological edema (e.g. in orbit or subcutaneous tissue) on T2 sequence, fat-supressed sequence such as STIR (short tau inversion recovery) is used, on which fat becomes dark and edema is hyperintense.

Table 3.2 Identification of MRI Sequences and Their Common Indications

Sequence	Ventricle	Other Features for Identification	Utility
T1	Hypointense	Gray matter – gray White matter – white	• Evaluation of anatomical details • Detection of hemorrhage • Assessing the degree of contrast enhancement on post-contrast images • Assessment of fat-containing lesions/structures
T2	Hyperintense	Gray matter – gray White matter – dark	• Detection of edema, tumor and most of the pathologies of brain
FLAIR	Hypointense	White matter being darker than gray matter Poor gray-white differentiation periventricular bright signal in older patients	• Lesions are better visualized as CSF and other non-pathological water signal is suppressed and only pathological edema is visualized
DWI	Hypointense	Poor gray-white differentiation	• Detection of cytotoxic edema (such as in acute infarcts) appears bright. • Abscess, epidermoid cyst, diffuse axonal injury
ADC	Hyperintense	Poor visualization of all anatomical details	• Restricted diffusion appears dark • Indications similar to DWI
T1 post-contrast	Hypointense	T1 with bright signal observed in vessels or patchy bright signal in meninges	• Tumor • Infective lesions
SWI	Hyperintense	Blooming artifacts near bone and temporal lobes Dark signal in basal ganglia and venous sinuses	• Detection of macro- and micro-hemorrhages • Calcification • Vascular malformations

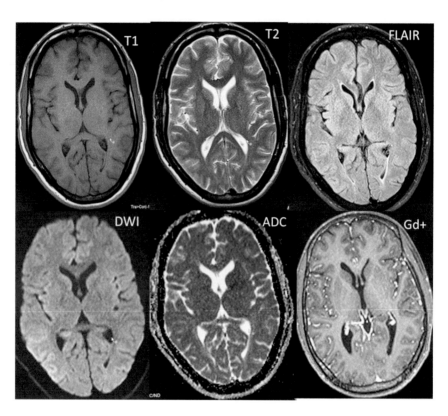

Figure 3.2 MRI images of same patient showing T1-weighted, T2-weighted, FLAIR (fluid-attenuated inversion recovery), DWI (diffusion-weighted image), ADC (apparent diffusion coefficient) map and Gd+ (post-gadolinium) contrast-enhanced images.

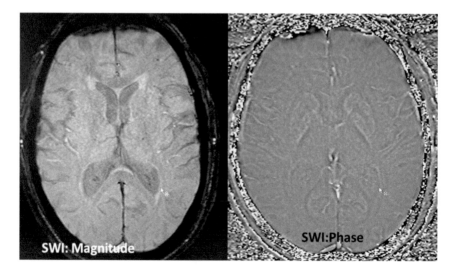

Figure 3.3 Susceptibility weighted images of a patient (magnitude and phase images).

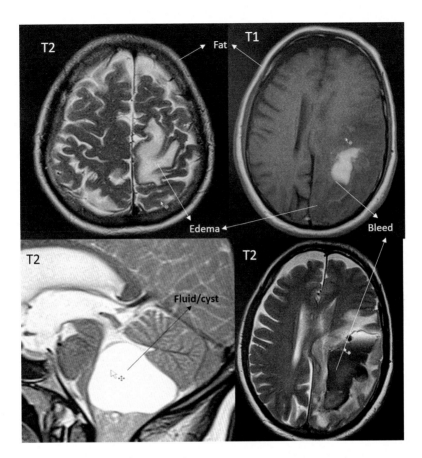

Figure 3.4 Characterization of various pathology on MRI sequences. Edema appears bright on T2 and dark on T1. Late subacute hemorrhage appearing bright on T1 and dark on T2. Fat (in subcutaneous tissue) is bright on both T1 and T2. Cyst appearing highly bright similar to ventricles.

- Calcification: dark on all sequences. Sometimes, they are difficult to detect on MRI. SWI/GRE can identify calcification with higher sensitivity.
- Fluid: fluid structures such as ventricles, CSF spaces, cysts, old infarct or bleed are highly bright on T2 and highly dark on T1. These are dark on FLAIR (suppression) and show facilitated diffusion (dark on DWI and bright on ADC). Notable exceptions are epidermoid cyst and brain abscesses, which show diffusion restriction.

Figure 3.4 illustrates the characterization of tissues and pathologies on MR sequences.

SYSTEMATIC INTERPRETATION OF CT HEAD

- *Bones*: use bone window and volume-rendered images to identify fractures and other bony focal lesions.

- *Extra-axial CSF spaces*: look for extradural/subdural/subarachnoid bleed/lesions. Use bone window to identify pneumocephalus.
- *Parenchyma and ventricles*: axial images:
  - Four lobes of brain and complete lateral ventricles and bilateral MCA cistern
  - Basal ganglia, internal capsule, thalami, external capsule and third ventricle
  - Brainstem
    - Midbrain and surrounding perimesencephalic cisterns
    - Pons and surrounding CSF space, cerebello-pontine angle and internal acoustic meatus
    - Medulla and surrounding CSF space
  - Cerebellum: bilateral cerebellar hemispheres, retrocerebellar regions, venous sinuses
- *Bilateral orbits*
- *Bilateral frontal, ethmoid, mastoid and sphenoid sinuses and bilateral mastoids*: bone window
- *Coronal images*: orbits, superior sagittal sinus, sellar-suprasellar region
- *Sagittal images*: sella, suprasellar region, pineal region, brainstem and fourth ventricle, cerebellar tonsils

MRI SEARCH PATTERN

On MRI similar search pattern remains the same as previously described for CT, however, the images are seen on each sequence.

- Start with axial FLAIR images, to identify bright lesions (edema/other pathology). Also evaluate extra-axial spaces for subdural/epidural bleed/lesions.
- Evaluate DWI and ADC, for areas of restricted diffusion.
- Evaluate T2 axial images for lesions that are T2 bright but may be iso to dark on FLAIR (FLAIR suppression). Also look for areas that are dark on T2.
- T1 images, for T1 bright areas in the parenchyma, ventricle and extra-axial CSF space that may represent bleed. T1 provides good anatomical detail, look for anatomical abnormalities, asymmetry.
- Post-contrast (T1) sequence: look for enhancing lesions and compare with T1 images.
- SWI should be seen for identification of microbleeds that can be missed on conventional sequences. If SWI or GRE is not done, b0 image of DWI should be seen.
- Following are the considerations to be looked for on MRI:
  - Whether the lesion is intra-axial (parenchymal) or extra-axial
  - What is the nature of lesion or signal change: edema/bleed/mass
  - Shape, extent and location of lesion
  - Mass effect produced by lesion
  - Correlate with clinical background

What are the important anatomical landmarks that one should remember?

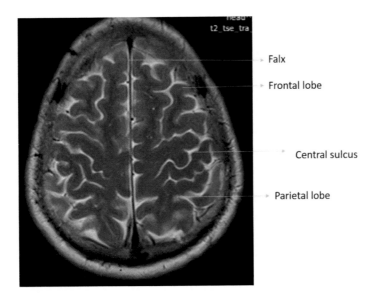

t2_tse_tra

→ Falx

→ Frontal lobe

Central sulcus

→ Parietal lobe

Figure 3.5 Axial T2W image showing superior aspect of cerebellar hemispheres.

- *Anatomy of cerebral hemisphere (identification of lobes)*
  - Interhemispheric fissure (contains falx): longitudinal cerebral fissure separates two hemispheres
  - Tentorium cerebelli: separates cerebrum and cerebellum
  - Frontal lobe is anterior to central sulcus and parietal lobe is posterior to it
  - Central (Rolandic) sulcus: it has a sigmoid hook shape (omega-shaped posterior bulge) (Figure 3.5)
  - Occipital lobe is posterior to parietooccipital sulcus. This sulcus is the deepest sulcus, perpendicular to interhemispheric fissure, inferiorly joins calcarine sulcus
  - Sylvian (lateral) fissure: separates frontal, temporal lobes anteriorly, courses laterally to cover insula
  - Temporal lobe occupies middle cranial fossa and is inferior to sylvian fissure. It contains amygdala (antero-superiorly) and hippocampus (postero-inferiorly) on the medial aspect
  - Insula: lies deep in the floor of sylvian fissure, overlapped by frontal, temporal, parietal "operculum"

- *Basal ganglia, thalamus and internal capsule* (Figure 3.6)
  - Caudate: along frontal horn of lateral ventricle (head) running along lateral ventricle
  - Anterior limb of internal capsule: capsule separates caudate head from lentiform nucleus

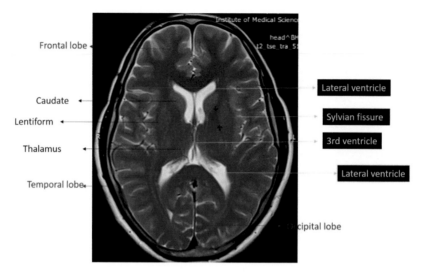

Figure 3.6 Axial T2W image showing basal ganglia, internal capsule (IC) and thalami.

- Lentiform nucleus: contains Galobus pallidus (medially) and Putamina (laterally)
- Posterior limb of internal capsule: separates thalamus from lentiform
- Thalamus: ovoid nucleus along both the lateral aspect of third ventricle, laterally bordered by internal capsule

- *Ventricle and cisterns (CSF spaces)*
  - Lateral ventricles: each has body, atrium (trigone), three horns (frontal, occipital and temporal horns)
  - Third ventricle: midline slit-like vertical cavity between bilateral thalami
  - Fourth ventricle: diamond-shaped cavity posterior to brainstem and anterior to cerebellum
  - Foramen of Monroe: communication between lateral ventricles and third ventricle
  - Aqueduct of sylvius: communication between third and fourth ventricle
  - Foramen of Magendie: midline posterior communication between fourth ventricle and retrocerebellar subarachnoid space
  - Foramen of Luschka: lateral communication between fourth ventricle and subarachnoid space (CP angle)

- *Brainstem: midbrain, pons and medulla (superior to inferior)* (Figures 3.7–3.9)
  - Midbrain
    - Cerebral peduncles: white matter tracts (corticospinal tract)
    - Tegmentum: anterior to aqueduct, contains substantia nigra and red nucleus

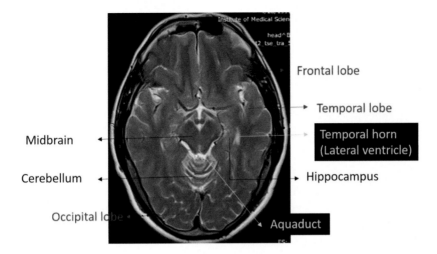

Figure 3.7 Axial T2W image showing lower aspect of cerebral hemisperes and midbrain.

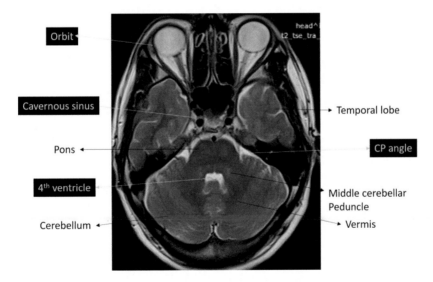

Figure 3.8 Axial T2W image showing cerebellar hemisperes and pons.

- – Tectum: superior and inferior colliculi
- – Adjacent CSF cisterns: interpeduncular (anterior), ambient (lateral), quadrigeminal plate (posterior)
- Pons
  - – Ventral (anterior) pons: white matter tracts
  - – Tegmentum (posterior)

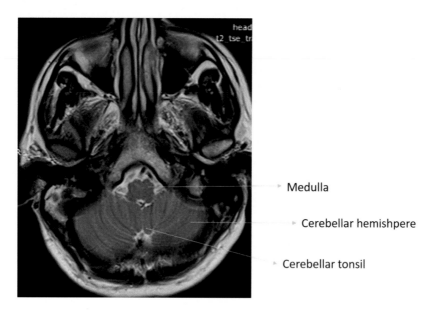

Figure 3.9 Axial T2W image showing cerebellar hemisperes and medulla.

- Cerebellopontine angle (CPA) cistern: lateral to pons and prepontine cistern (anterior to pons)
- Medulla
  - Ventral (anterior) medulla: olive and pyramidal tract (corticospinal tract)
  - Tegmentum (posterior): white matter
  - Premedullary cistern (anterior to medulla)

- *Cerebellum: located posterior to brainstem and fourth ventricle*
  - Two hemispheres and midline vermis
  - Superior cerebellar peduncle: connects cerebellum to midbrain
  - Middle cerebellar peduncle: connects to pons
  - Inferior cerebellar peduncle: connects to medulla

- *Sella, pituitary and cavernous sinus* (Figure 3.10)
  - Sella: concave midline depression in sphenoid; anteriorly, tuberculum sellae and anterior clinoid processes; posteriorly, dorsum sellae, posterior clinoid processes; superiorly: suprasellar cistern, optic chiasma and hypothalamus
  - Pituitary: larger anterior pituitary (T1 isointense to brain) and posterior pituitary (T1 hyperintense)
  - Cavernous sinus: paired septated, dural-lined venous sinuses lateral to suprasellar cistern, also contains internal cerebral arteries and cranial nerves 3,4,5,6

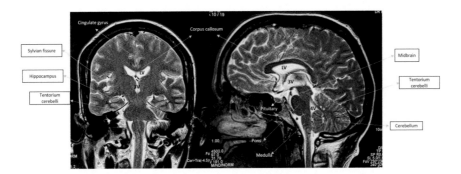

Figure 3.10 T2 coronal and sagittal images of brain.

IMAGING CONSIDERATIONS IN TRAUMATIC HEAD INJURY

Choice of imaging: non-contrast CT

Indication of imaging (New Orleans criteria): loss of consciousness, GCS 15, normal neurological examination with any of the following: headache, vomiting, age > 60 years, alcohol intoxication, short-term memory loss, seizure, physical evidence of trauma in head and neck

Indication for repeat CT: any patient with neurological deterioration and routine repeat CT may be warranted among patients with GCS < 9

Indication of MRI (to detect diffuse axonal injury): loss of consciousness persisting greater than six hours after injury, no hemorrhage on CT.

Positive CT findings (New Orleans criteria)

- Skull fractures (depressed)
- Cerebral contusion: hemorrhage in cortex
- Parenchymal hematoma (Figure 3.11)
- Epidural hematoma: hyperdense biconvex collection that don't cross suture (may cross falx/tentorium) (Figure 3.11)
- Subdural hematoma: crescent-shaped collection that don't cross Falx/tentorium, may cross sutures
- Subarachnoid hemorrhage: hyperdensity within sulci/cisterns. Hyperdense contents in ventricle suggest intraventricular hemorrhage

Mass effect should be noted in form of effacement of ventricles, hydrocephalus and transcompartmental herniation (Figure 3.12):

- Subfalcine herniation
- Descending transtentorial herniation
- Uncal herniation
- Ascending transtentorial herniation
- Tonsillar herniation into spinal canal

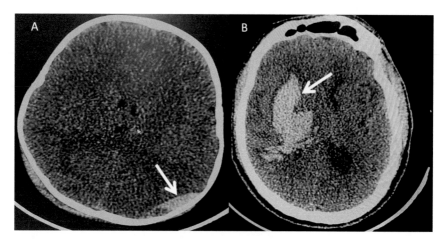

Figure 3.11 (A) NCCT images showing biconvex extradural hematoma in left parietal region (*arrow*) and (B) acute intraparenchyma traumatic hemorrhage in right basal ganglia, thalamus, internal capsule (*arrow*).

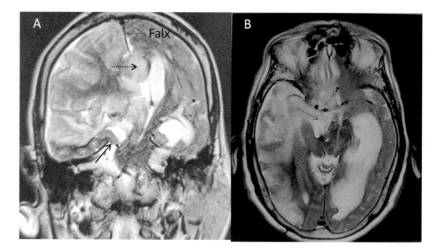

Figure 3.12 Coronal (A) T2-weighted image of a patient with a large right cerebral infarct with edema shows mass effect in form of right to left subfalcine (*dotted arrow*) and right descending transtentorial (*arrow*) hernia; (B) T2 axial image of same patient showing right uncus herniation (*arrow*).

IMAGING CONSIDERATIONS IN ACUTE STROKE

- Acute stroke patients who are candidates for IV thrombolysis (0–4.5-hour window), either non-contrast CT of the brain are recommended to exclude intracranial hemorrhage and determine the extent of ischemic changes. CT is usually preferred because it can be done more timely, although MRI is more sensitive.

- Alberta Stroke Program Early CT Score (ASPECTS), a simple 10-point pre-treatment non-contrast CT score that divides the MCA territory into 10 regions and identifies patients with stroke who are unlikely to have good outcome from thrombolysis.
- CT angiography/MR angiography of neck and brain used to evaluate cause of stroke: identify thrombus, guide intra-arterial thrombolysis or clot retrieval, evaluation of the carotid and vertebral arteries in the neck, establishing stroke aetiology (e.g. atherosclerosis, dissection, web).
- CT perfusion: identification of infarct core and ischemic penumbra that can be salvaged.
- Imaging findings in infarct (Figure 3.13). Table 3.3 summarizes the imaging findings in infarcts.

INTRACEREBRAL HEMORRHAGE

- Occurs in 10% of strokes and is a leading cause of death and disability in adults. Important causes of spontaneous intracranial hemorrhage are hypertension, cerebral amyloid angiopathy, aneurysms, vascular malformations and hemorrhagic infarcts (both venous and arterial).
- *Intraparenchymal hemorrhage* can be of three types. Centrally located hemorrhage (basal ganglia, pons or cerebellum) is caused by hypertension. Lobar hemorrhage (periphery of a lobe) can be seen in cerebral amyloid angiopathy. Microbleeds is caused due to chronic hypertension, amyloid angiopathy or vasculitis.
- NCCT is the first-line modality to diagnose bleed where it is seen as an irregular hyperdense lesion in parenchyma with surrounding edema. Mass effect can be seen as effacement of sulci, ventricles and herniation.
- MR with gradient-recalled echo (GRE) imaging, susceptibility-weighted imaging (SWI) are sensitive to hemorrhage. MR with MR angiography [MRA], MR venography [MRV], performed following CT to assess the cause of hemorrhage.

MR imaging appearance of bleed (Figure 3.14): Table 3.4 *summarizes the MRI findings in CNS bleeds.*

- Extra-axial hemorrhage: subarachnoid hemorrhage (along sulci, MCA or sylvian fissure), cisternal bleed or intraventicular bleed. NCCT is the modality of choice. CT angiography should be done to look for aneurysm if SAH is present (Figure 3.15). Digital subtraction angiography (DSA) is the gold standard for diagnosis and characterization of aneurysms and other vascular abnormalities.
- CT scan is sensitive for detection of SAH, however, sensitivity of CT is thought to decline with the passage of time, and lumbar puncture is still recommended.

Table 3.3 Imaging Findings for Cerebral Infarcts

Stage	NCCT	T1	T2/FLAIR	DWI/ADC	Others
Immediate	Hyperdense MCA	Normal	Normal Loss of flow void	Restriction	Occlusion on CTA/MRA
Early hyperacute	Loss of gray-white differentiation Hypodense lentiform Insular ribbon	Normal	Normal Loss of flow void	Restriction	Occlusion on CTA/MRA
Late hyperacute (> 6 hours)	Loss of gray-white differentiation Hypodense lentiform Insular ribbon	Hypointensity (after 16 hours)	Bright signal	Restriction	Occlusion on CTA/MRA
Acute (first week)	Significant edema with mass effect	Hypointense Cortex hyperintensity (after 3 days)	Hyperintense (progressive increase in signal till 4 days)	Restriction ADC starts increasing at end of first week	T1 contrast images: cortical enhancement (5 days) Arterial enhancement Meningeal enhancement
Subacute (10–15 days)	CT fogging: cortical petechial bleed Normal cortex	Hypointense Cortex hyperintense (laminar necrosis)	Hyperintense T2 fogging (2 weeks)	ADC pseudo normalization DWI bright (T2 shine through)	T1 contrast images: cortical enhancement
Chronic	Gliosis, negative mass effect, cystic changes, hyperdense cortex	High T1 in the cortex	Hyperintense	High ADC Variable DWI	Cortical enhancement (2–4 months) *Consider mass in enhancement > 12 weeks

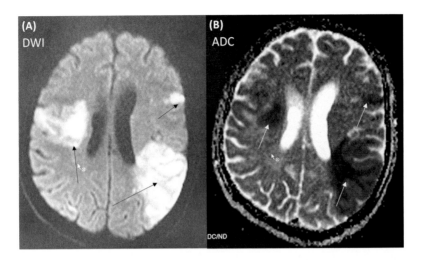

Figure 3.13 (A) Diffusion-weighted images and (B) ADC map showing multiple areas of restricted diffusion in bilateral cerebral hemispheres (*arrows*) suggestive of acute infarcts.

Table 3.4 MRI Appearances for CNS Bleeds

Bleed	Component	T1W	T2W
Hyperacute (<12 h)	Intracellular oxyhemoglobin	Iso	Bright
Acute (hours to days)	Intracellular deoxyhemoglobin	Iso	Dark
Early Subacute (few days)	Intracellular methemoglobin	Bright	Dark
Late Subacute (weeks to months)	Extracellular methemoglobin	Bright	Bright
Chronic	Hemosiderin	Dark	Dark

OTHER ACUTE NEUROLOGICAL CONDITIONS, DIFFERENTIALS AND IMAGING CONSIDERATIONS

Brain death in coma patients

Brain death is characterized by diffuse cerebral edema with effacement of the gray-white matter differentiation and hyperdense cerebellum (reversal or white cerebellum sign). CT/MR angiography shows non-opacification/non-visualization of the middle cerebral arteries and intracranial vessels.

Headache

Differential considerations are subarachnoid hemorrhage (SAH), hydrocephalus, mass, infective lesions venous thrombosis. NCCT should be performed first and

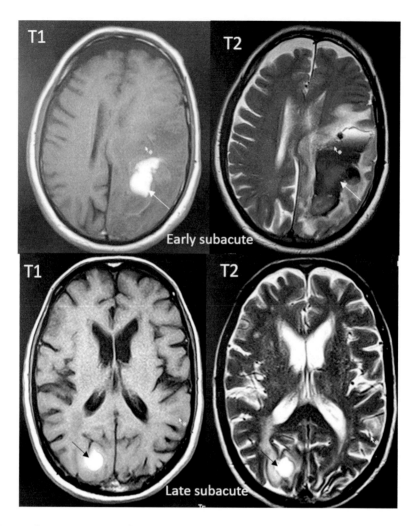

Figure 3.14 (A,B) T1- and T2-weighted images of early subacute parenchymal hemorrhage showing T1 hyperintense and T2 hypointense area in left parieral lobe. (C,D) T1- and T2-weighted images of late subacute parenchymal hemorrhage showing T1 hyperintense and T2 hyperintense area in right occipital lobe.

subsequently MRI, CECT or CT/MR venography/angiography should be done depending on the findings.

Seizures

Infective lesions (neurocysticercosis, tuberculomas, meningitis), mass, mesial temporal sclerosis (Figure 3.16), cortical abnormalities can cause seizures. Contrast-enhanced CT and preferably MRI with contrast should be done. MRI protocol should include Coronal FLAIR and 3D T1 sequences.

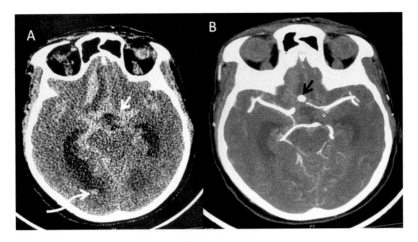

Figure 3.15 (A) NCCT image showing extensive subarachnoid hemorrhage (*short arrow*) in basal cisterns and intraventricular hemorrhage (*curved arrow*). (B) CT angiography of the same patient showing aneurysm (*black arrow*) arising from anterior communicating artery.

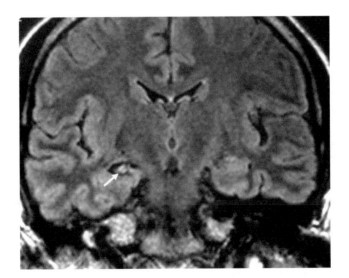

Figure 3.16 Coronal FLAIR image of a patient with seizures showing atrophic and hyperintense right hippocampus (*arrow*) suggestive of mesial temporal sclerosis.

Fever

Infective lesions should be suspected. CECT or preferably contrast MRI can be done.

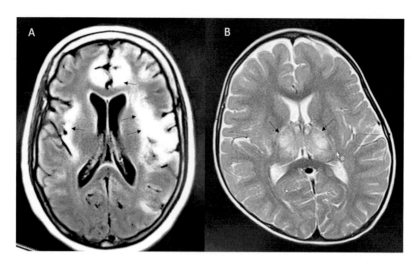

Figure 3.17 (A) FLAIR axial image in a patient with fever and altered sensorium showing hyperintense area in bilateral temporal and bilateral frontal lobes suggestive of HSV encephalitis. (B) Axial T2-weighted image of a patient with Japanese encephalitis showing T2 hyperintensities in bilateral thalami (arrows) and putamina.

Table 3.5 Differential Diagnosis of Ring-Enhancing Lesions and Differential of Basal Ganglia/Thalamic Lesions (Common)

Ring-enhancing Lesion	Basal Ganglia and Thalamic Lesions
Abscess (pyogenic/fungal/ tubercular)	Japanese encephalitis
Tuberculoma	Toxicity (methanol/carbon monoxide/ organophosphate)
Neurocysticercosis	Metabolic (osmotic myelinolysis/hepatic encephalopathy/uremic encephalopathy/
Metastasis	hypoxic ischemic encephalopathy)
Glioblastoma	Neurodegenerative (Wilson disease, mitochondrial, Creutzfeldt-Jakob disease, Huntington/autoimmune encephalitis)

Classically, it was thought that encephalitis (viral infection) affects the cortex and cerebritis (bacterial infection) affects white matter, but overlap exists. HSV encephalitis presents as a hypodense signal in the insular cortex initially and then extends to the entire temporal lobe, bilateral frontal lobe and contralateral temporal lobe (Figure 3.17a). Japanese encephalitis presents with T2/FLAIR hyperintensity in bilateral basal ganglia and thalami (hypodense on CT) (Figure 3.17b) (Table 3.5). Cerebritis can be seen as an ill-defined area of edema (hypodense on CT, hyperintense on T2/FLAIR) in cortical and subcortical. Cerebritis can progress to brain abscess if untreated, which can be seen as ring-enhancing lesion on

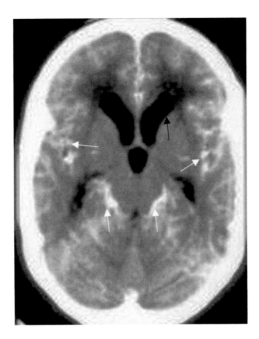

Figure 3.18 Axial CT contrast-enhanced CT (CECT) image of a patient with tubercular meningitis showing extensive leptomeningeal thickening (*white arrows*) and hydrocephalus (*black arrow*).

CECT and contrast MRI. The central non-enhancing component of abscess shows diffusion restriction. Meningitis is seen as leptomeningeal enhancement (enhancing tissue in the subarachnoid space) in basal cisterns, along the sulci, around middle cerebral artery, which may be associated with hydrocephalus (Figure 3.18). Subdural empyema can be seen as crescentic extra-axial collection with enhancing meningeal lining.

Key points

- A study suggested interpretation of a non-contrast head CT takes an average of 39 minutes with the help of a teleradiology support system, potentially wasting precious time in patients with intracranial hemorrhage or ischemic stroke. Hence, the ability of the emergency physician to interpret the CT could be extremely valuable.
- *What is the role of digital subtraction angiography (DSA) and interventional radiology in the management of neurological emergencies?*
  - Diagnosis of occult aneurysm not visible on CTA/MRA and coiling of aneurysm
  - Intra-arterial injection of tPA (within 6 hours)
  - Arteriovenous malformation embolization
  - Cerebral tumor embolization
  - Carotid angioplasty/stenting

4

Locomotor system

VAISHALI UPADHYAY, KHUSHBOO PILANIA
AND ANIRBAN HOM CHOUDHURI

INTRODUCTION

Both traumatic and nontraumatic emergencies can involve the locomotor system (musculoskeletal system) and can be witnessed in the ICU. Some musculoskeletal complications are iatrogenic in nature while some occur after a prolonged ICU and hospital stay.

Imaging plays a pivotal role in the diagnosis and management of such disorders because clinical examination and diagnosis is grossly limited owing to altered mentation and poor comprehensibility.

The common conditions are:

- Traumatic injuries of the spine, thorax and pelvis
- Medical complications such as diabetic myonecrosis, rhabdomyolysis
- Disuse atrophy of nerves and muscles
- Critical illness–induced polyneuropathy and myopathy
- Drug-induced myopathies viz. steroids, antimalarials, anti-HIV etc.

AIM OF IMAGING

a. To confirm clinical diagnosis
b. To measure the severity and extent of the injury or disease
c. Early detection of potential complications such as vascular or visceral injuries, compartment syndrome etc.

IMAGING MODALITIES

We shall limit ourselves to the key modalities useful in everyday practice.

 DOI: 10.1201/9781003218739-4

Bedside X-ray

- Preferred modality for initial screening
- Cost effective and widely available
- Optimum for evaluation of bony injuries
- Detection of osteomyelitis

Bedside USG

- Done using curvilinear and high-frequency (5–20 MHz) linear transducers
- Cost effective and widely available
- No radiation hazard and hence can be repeated frequently, if indicated
- High spatial resolution
- Can be done in any position
- Not contraindicated in pregnant patients
- Both static and dynamic assessment are possible
- Good to visualize superficial structures such as muscles and tendons
- Good to assess vascular injuries and associated complications
- Useful to guide bedside interventions
- Operator dependent
- Difficult to evaluate deep-seated structures or those which are underneath bones
- Usefulness is impaired in the presence of scarring or calcification

CT Scan

- High spatial resolution
- Rapid scanning
- Better than X-ray in detecting fractures and bony complications
- Not performed bedside and hence less preferred in ICU patients with limited mobility
- Costly
- Greater radiation exposure
- Contraindicated during pregnancy to avoid fetal damage

MRI

- Multiplanar imaging modality
- High contrast resolution
- No radiation exposure
- Can be performed after the first trimester in pregnant patients
- Most sensitive modality for assessment of spinal cord injuries and hematomas
- Expensive
- Less widely available
- Less preferred in ICU patients when transportation is difficult and risky

- Increased scan time
- Contraindicated in patients with pacemakers, cochlear implants etc.
- Difficult in claustrophobic patients
- Prone to motion artefacts
- Limited usefulness in the presence of metallic substances

CARDINAL TECHNICAL POINTERS

Imaging in muscle pathologies

MYOPATHIES, RHABDOMYOLYSIS AND POLYMYOSITIS

- Myositis/myopathy, rhabdomyolysis and polymyositis are among the common acute muscular disorders seen in the ICU.
- Imaging supports their diagnosis, delineates sites for biopsy and also guides therapy.
- MRI is the modality of choice in most muscle disorders, though in ICU USG has greater feasibility.

- *USG*
  - Myopathies are seen as diffuse altered echogenicity of the muscles, which appear hypoechoic in cases with predominant edema and hyperechoic when fatty infiltration sets in (Figure 4.1).

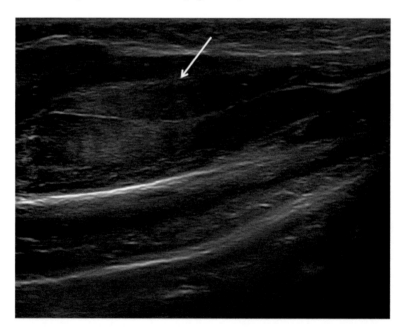

Figure 4.1 Longitudinal axis USG image of a child with sepsis and tenderness in left leg showing edema in the muscles of the posterior compartment consistent with myositis.

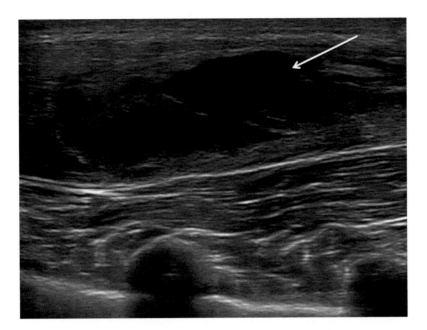

Figure 4.2 Longitudinal axis USG image of an adult male with tenderness in right paraspinal region showing a hypoechoic collection with internal septa and debris in right erector spinae muscle, suggestive of pyomyositis.

- In rhabdomyolysis, apart from reduced echogenicity, the muscles have a hazy and cloudy echotexture with architectural distortion and fascial thickening. There are also interspersed hyperechoic and peripheral non-vascular anechoic areas.
- Pyomyositis has an appearance similar to rhabdomyolysis, but there are more often intramuscular hypoechoic collections with intense peripheral vascularity due to increased inflammation (Figures 4.2 and 4.3).

- *On MRI*
  - Myopathies are seen as multifocal muscle edema and atrophy usually with a symmetric distribution (Figure 4.4).
  - In rhabdomyolysis, the affected muscles show edema and geographical areas of altered signal and heterogenous rim-like pattern of enhancement on contrast study (Figure 4.5a, b).
  - In pyomyositis, there is muscle edema in the initial stage which appears T1 hypointense and T2 hyperintense. Subsequently, abscess formation occurs. An abscess shows low to intermediate signal intensity on T1 images and appears hyperintense on T2 images with extensive surrounding edema. Post-contrast fat-suppressed T1 images show peripheral enhancement (Figure 4.6a–c).

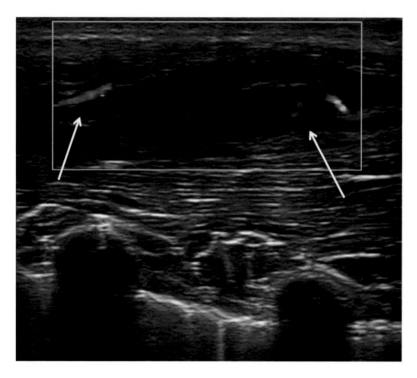

Figure 4.3 Longitudinal axis color Doppler image of the same patient as in Figure 4.2, showing increased peripheral vascularity in the lesion.

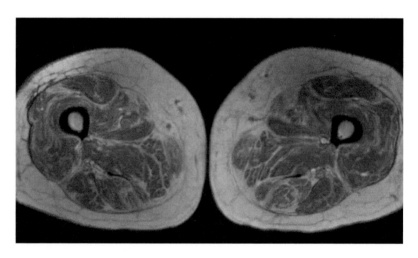

Figure 4.4 Axial T1W MR image of the thighs showing bilaterally symmetrical atrophy of muscles of all the compartments consistent with chronic myopathy in a patient after a prolonged ICU stay.

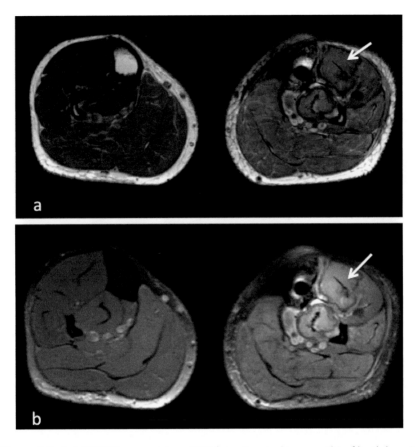

Figure 4.5 Axial T2W images (a) and PD fat-saturated images (b) of both legs in a young male patient who underwent surgery for fractures of left tibia and fibula showing altered signal intensity in the muscles of the anterior compartment and tibialis posterior on left side (*white arrows*) with curvilinear intramuscular T2 hypointensities, consistent with rhabdomyolysis.

DIAPHRAGMATIC MUSCLE DYSFUNCTION

- Leads to progressive deterioration of the respiratory status.
- Can occur in ICU patients due to critical illness myopathy, ventilator use, or due to phrenic nerve injury from chest support devices or tube placement.
- In recent times, often seen in critically ill COVID-19 patients.
- Fluoroscopy sniff test is a quick and real-time assessment of diaphragm excursion.
- *Role of USG in diaphragmatic muscle dysfunction:*
  - Detecting presence or absence of diaphragm muscle atrophy
  - Calculating muscle thickening ratio with respiration
  - Evaluation of excursion with M mode imaging

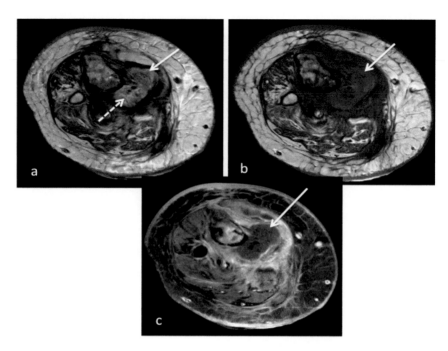

Figure 4.6 Axial T2W image (a), T1W image (b) and post-contrast fat-saturated T1W image (c) of the left leg in a 56-year-old female showing a thick peripherally enhancing T1 hypointense and T2 hyperintense collection (*white arrows*), suggestive of abscess. Few interspersed air foci (*dashed arrow in a*) are seen within it.

LONG-TERM MUSCULAR SEQUELAE IN ICU PATIENTS

Muscle wasting [sarcopenia and cachexia] is one of the greatest problems in ICU survivors and is associated with the extent of organ failure and duration of length of stay.

- *USG*
  - Quantitative assessment of muscle can be done – based on muscle layer thickness and cross-sectional area of an individual muscle or muscle group.
  - Qualitative assessment of muscle can be done – based on muscle echogenicity.
  - Limitations include heterogeneity in parameters measured and reported and interindividual variability in muscle size.

- *MRI*
  - The muscles show decreased size with fat infiltration.
  - Often difficult to transport the patient from the ICU to the MRI scan room.

Imaging in pathologies of the skin and subcutaneous tissues

- Cellulitis, necrotizing fasciitis, abscesses and hematomas can be seen in patients in the ICU set-up. These conditions can be easily diagnosed with USG performed using high-frequency linear transducer.
- USG can also be used for aspiration in these conditions.

- *USG*
    - Cellulitis has a "cobblestone" appearance in which echogenic subcutaneous fat lobules are separated by hypoechoic fluid-filled areas (Figure 4.7). There is increased echogenicity of the skin. Increased vascularity of the affected areas is seen on color Doppler.
    - In necrotizing fasciitis, there is fascial thickening with fluid collections, extensive involvement of both peripheral and deep intermuscular fascia, involvement of three or more compartments and associated subcutaneous edema. Air can be seen in the soft tissues as echogenic foci with posterior dirty shadowing.
    - Abscesses are seen as hypoechoic collections within the infected soft tissue. Peripheral vascularity is increased. Adjacent subcutaneous edema is seen. Extent of liquefaction within the abscess depends on the maturity of the abscess, and the volume of the same can be detected with USG.
    - Hematomas are often indistinguishable from abscesses on USG, though the peripheral vascularity on color Doppler in cases of abscesses is much higher (Figure 4.8).

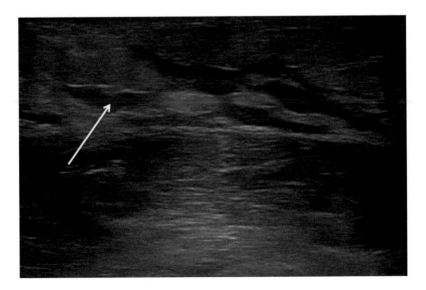

Figure 4.7 Longitudinal axis USG image in an elderly female patient with cellulitis in left arm showing "cobblestone" appearance in the subcutaneous fat plane.

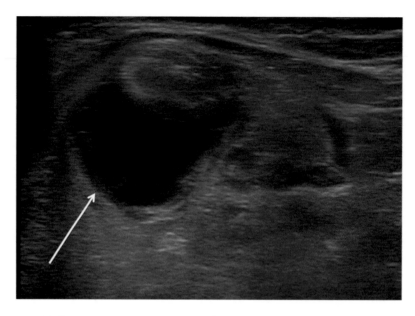

Figure 4.8 Transverse axis USG image of an adult male patient with a contained haematoma in the right upper thigh after femoral artery cannulation.

Imaging in nerve injuries/neuropathies

- These may be the indication for the ICU admission but may develop secondary to a stay in the ICU.
- Electrophysiological tests such as EMG and NCV have been traditionally used for evaluation of nerves, but they have limited ability to delineate the site and severity of neural damage.
- High-resolution USG and MRI including MR neurography have emerged as excellent modalities to assess the site, extent and severity of damage to the nerve.
- Normal peripheral nerves have a honeycomb appearance on USG due to the presence of hypoechoic fascicles surrounded by echogenic connective tissue. On MRI, nerves appear isointense to muscle in T1 images and isointense to mildly hyperintense in T2 images.
- On USG, abnormal nerves appear hypoechoic, and on MRI, they show increased T2 signal. There is also nerve enlargement with loss of fascicular architecture depending on the severity of insult.

PERIPHERAL NERVES

- Traumatic injuries
- Iatrogenic injuries: there has been an increased incidence of such injuries in patients admitted with COVID-19 in the ICU. The postulated mechanisms have been increased vulnerability of the nerves due to the hyperinflammatory

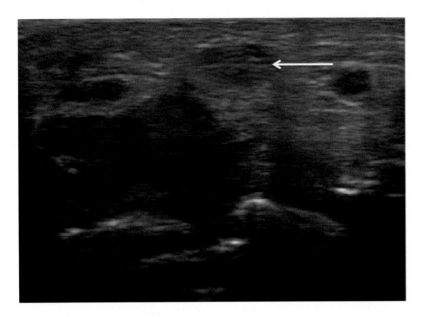

Figure 4.9 Transverse axis USG image in a patient with COVID-19 infection and clinical median neuropathy showing thickened hypoechoic median nerve.

state and increased need of proning to maintain oxygen levels, which lead to stretching and compression injuries. Most of the COVID-19-related nerve injuries are due to axonotmesis.

- *USG and MRI in nerve injuries*
  - Help in grading the severity of nerve injury, as per Seddon and Sunderland classifications, and differentiating neuropraxia from axonotmesis and neurotmesis.
  - Neuropraxic injury: seen as a change in the echogenicity/signal intensity of the involved nerve but without any focal change in calibre.
  - Axonotmesis: focal segment of the nerve showing calibre change and enlarged fascicles or effacement of the normal fascicular pattern (Figure 4.9). The nerve continuity is maintained, however.
  - Neurotmesis: focal discontinuity of the nerve. Exact assessment of the length of the gap between fibres and the appearance of the nerve fibres at the torn end is important for surgical planning.
  - Intraneural foreign bodies can be easily localized with USG.
  - Extrinsic compression of the nerve due to haematoma can be seen.
  - Secondary muscle denervation is seen in the form of muscle edema in early phases and atrophy with fatty infiltration in the chronic setting.

- *Chronic inflammatory demyelinating polyneuropathy*: involves the peripheral nerves in a symmetrical fashion with the nerves appearing thickened on both USG and MRI. Contrast enhancement is usually not present.

- *Post-infectious peripheral neuropathy*: when this occurs in the brachial plexus, it is known as Parsonage-Turner syndrome. MR neurography reveals unilateral or bilaterally asymmetrical enlarged nerves of the brachial plexus with T2 hyperintense signal and associated denervation changes in muscles.
- *Critical illness polyneuropathy*: a symmetric sensorimotor axonal polyneuropathy that develops in patients with prolonged hospitalization and ICU stay.

SPINAL CORD AND INTRA-SPINAL NERVES

MRI is the preferred imaging modality for evaluation of lesions of the spinal cord and intra-spinal nerves. These include cord injury, Guillain-Barre syndrome (GBS) and myelitis.

- *Cord injury*: the site, extent and severity are seen well on MRI.
  - In cord edema, there is a T1 normal/hypointense signal and a T2 hyperintense signal, which may be associated with cord swelling (Figure 4.10a).

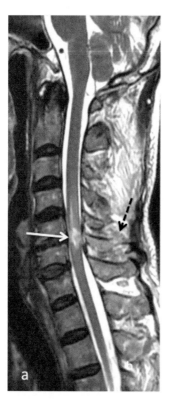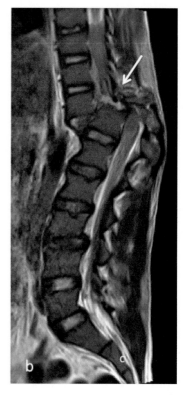

Figure 4.10 Sagittal T2W image of the cervical spine (a) in a patient with road traffic accident showing T2 hyperintense lesion in the cord opposite C5–6 level, consistent with non-hemorrhagic cord contusion. Also noted is fracture of the spinous process (*black dashed arrow*, a). Sagittal T2W image of the dorso-lumbar spine (b) in another patient with severe spinal injury showing cord transection at D11–12 level.

- Hemorrhagic cord contusion (<4 mm) and cord haematoma (>4 mm) are seen as T2 hypointense lesions with hyperintense rim. These lesions are best visualized on GRE T2 images.
- Cord transection is seen as a complete loss of continuity in the spinal cord (Figure 4.10b).
- Cord compression can occur due to displaced vertebral fracture fragments or associated haematoma. The cord contour is deformed at the site of compression, and there can be associated changes in signal intensity.

- *GBS*: thickening and enhancement of the cauda equina nerve roots is seen. MRI is usually done in these cases to rule out any other proximal cord pathology.
- *Myelitis*: seen as signal alteration involving a long/short segment of the cord. These changes in signal intensity are T2 hyperintense (Figure 4.11a, b). Contrast enhancement may or may not be present. There is preferential involvement of the thoracic cord.
- *Epidural haematoma*: may result in paraparesis in patients on blood thinners or patients with coagulopathy. In the majority of cases, the haematoma is seen posteriorly or posterolaterally in the spinal canal. It can show variable

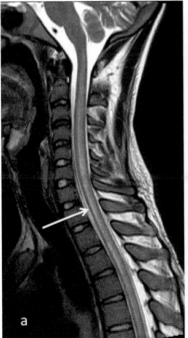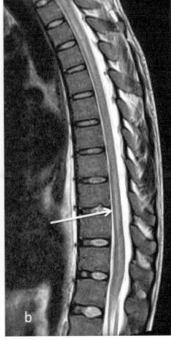

Figure 4.11 Sagittal T2W images of the cervico-dorsal spine (a) and dorsal spine (b) in a young female patient with quadriparesis following fever showing extensive T2 hyperintense signal in the spinal cord, consistent with myelitis.

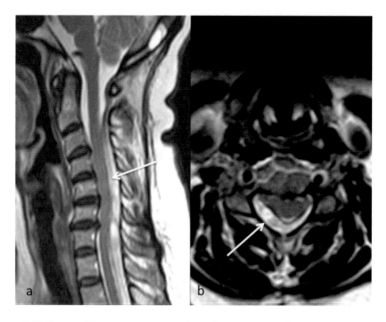

Figure 4.12 Sagittal T2W image (a) and axial T2W image (b) showing a posterior epidural haematoma extending from C2 to D5 level, which is causing mild cord compression.

hypo- to hyperintense signal on T1 and T2 images depending on the stage of blood degradation products. There is compression of the thecal sac at the level of the haematoma and effacement of the epidural fat (Figure 4.12a, b).

Imaging in spinal trauma

- Clinical evaluation and information on the nature of trauma are the most important factors to decide if imaging is needed and the type of imaging modality.
- Imaging is needed especially for unstable lesions that can be responsible for serious neurologic complications.
- Stable and alert patients who fulfil the Canadian C-Spine Rule or the NEXUS low-risk criteria may not be imaged.
- Role of imaging in spinal trauma:
  - To diagnose and characterize the type of injury
  - To estimate the severity of injury
  - To assess for potential spinal instability
  - To evaluate the status of the spinal cord and surrounding structures (MRI is the gold standard technique)

The role of different imaging modalities has been discussed in the subsequent sections.

RADIOGRAPHS

- These are the first line of imaging in most cases of spinal trauma.
- Minimal radiographic assessment for spine consists of anteroposterior and lateral views. In cases of cervical spine, additional odontoid/open-mouth view is mandatory.
- The lateral view is the most important radiograph to acquire. In cervical spine, the cervicothoracic junction must be seen as supplemented by additional views (swimmer's or oblique views) or by gently pulling down the shoulders.
- Flexion-extension radiographs are important optional views to diagnose atlantoaxial instability.
- The severity of the injury depends on:
  - Fracture morphology (compression, distraction, rotation/translation)
  - Integrity of the discoligamentous complex
  - The patient's neurologic status

- For cervical spine injury, the ABC method, proposed by Daffner and Harris, is used.
  - Alignment
    - Lateral view: the anterior and posterior vertebral lines, the spinolaminar and interspinous lines should be assessed for continuity.
    - AP view: spinous processes should be in midline and regularly spaced.
    - Odontoid view: lateral masses should be aligned.
  - Bone integrity: maintained vertebral body height and no fracture line
  - Cartilage (joints): "rule of twos" – the interlaminar (interspinous) space, interpedicle distance (transverse or vertical), unilateral or bilateral atlantoaxial offset, and the interfacetal joint width must not differ by > 2 mm. *The interlaminar distance is more reliable and accurate than the interspinous distance to explore hyperflexion injuries.*
  - Soft tissue: retropharyngeal thickness
    - At C2 level should not be more than 7 mm (both children and adults).
    - At C6 level should not be more than 14 mm (in children) or 22 mm (in adults).

- Other important measurements especially for craniovertebral junction
  - BDI: basion-dental interval should not be more than 12 mm in adults or children > 13 years.
  - BAI: basion-axial interval should be between + 12 mm and – 4 mm.
  - Normal ADI is < 3 mm in adults and < 5 mm in children, and a larger distance reflects a high probability of ligamentous injury [atlantoaxial anteroposterior dislocation].

- Various specific injuries are encountered at the craniovertebral junction
  - Occipital condyle fractures
  - Occipitoatlantal dislocation
    - Assessed with the BDI-BAI (Harris's method) described previously.

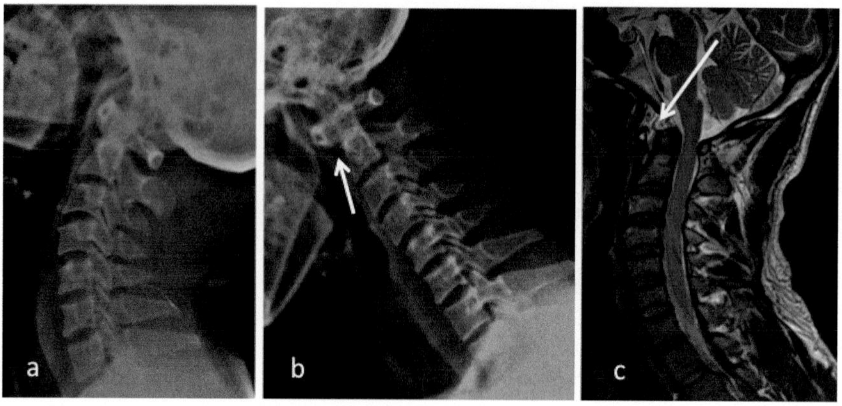

Figure 4.13 Lateral radiographs of the cervical spine in extension (a), flexion (b) and sagittal T2W MR image (c) of a patient with post-traumatic atlantoaxial dislocation.

  – Powers' ratio-basion-posterior atlas arch distance/opisthion-anterior arch distance. Values > 1 are pathologic.
  – X-line method: pathologic if the line from basion to the axis spinolaminar junction does not intersect C2 or if a line from the opisthion to the posteroinferior corner of the body of the axis does not intersect C1.
- Atlas fractures
- Odontoid process/dens fracture
- Hangman's fracture: fracture of both pars interarticularis of C2
- Atlantoaxial anteroposterior dislocation/atlantoaxial rotary subluxation (Figure 4.13a–c)

CT SCAN

- It is being increasingly advocated for unconscious patients not meeting low-risk criteria. It enables excellent depiction of fractures and displaced fracture fragments, especially with coronal, sagittal and 3D reconstructions (Figures 4.14a–d, 4.15a–d).
- CT angiogram may be needed to assess the integrity and relationship of the major vessels to the site of injury. It is also often needed to determine the location of the vertebral artery prior to posterior instrumentation procedures.

MRI

- It is the only modality to assess the status of the spinal cord in cases with neurologic symptoms where spinal cord compression or injury is suspected (Figure 4.16a, b).
- It is the only imaging modality that can detect the pathology in SCIWORA (spinal cord injury without radiographic abnormality). These injuries are typically located in the cervical region and should be suspected in patients with blunt trauma with early symptoms of neurologic deficit.

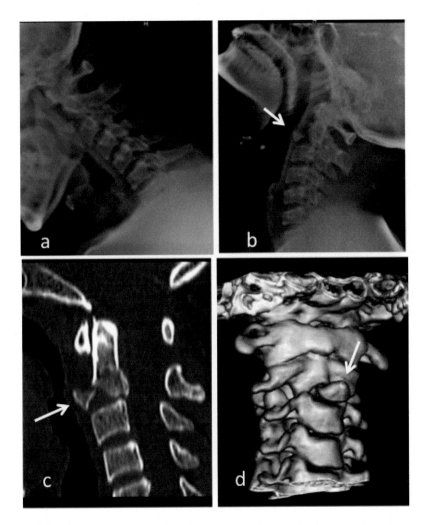

Figure 4.14 Lateral radiographs of the cervical spine in flexion (a), extension (b), sagittal reformatted CT image (c) and 3D reconstructed CT image (d) in a patient with fracture of the C2 vertebral body with anteriorly displaced fracture fragment.

- There should be a low threshold for MRI in paediatric patients as spinal cord injuries without radiographic abnormality (SCIWORA) are more common in the paediatric age group.
- MRI is also helpful in assessment of ligament/muscle injury such as the status of the posterior ligamentous complex in cases of burst fracture, which is a critical determinant of surgical indication.
- It is the problem-solving tool in cases of discordance between clinical status and CT imaging.

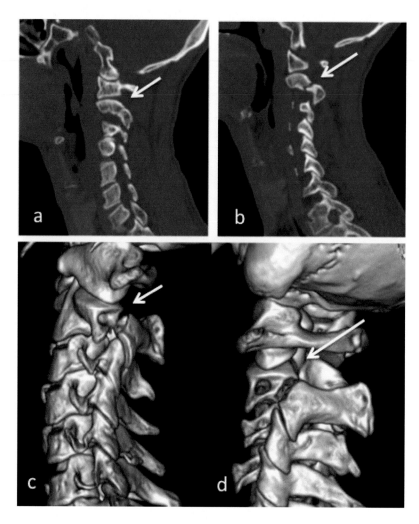

Figure 4.15 Lateral radiographs of the cervical spine (a and b) and 3D reconstructed CT images (c and d) in a patient with hangman's fracture showing fracture of bilateral pars interarticularis of C2.

FREQUENTLY ASKED QUESTIONS

Q1. Which modality is most useful in evaluation of rhabdomyolysis?

Answer: MRI has increased sensitivity as compared to USG and CT scan in the detection of rhabdomyolysis. It can accurately identify the distribution and extent of the involved muscles by detecting changes in their signal intensity. Imaging findings have to be correlated with clinical and laboratory parameters to establish the diagnosis.

Q2. What is MR neurography?

Answer: MR neurography includes a combination of two-dimensional and three-dimensional T1W and T2W sequences with fat suppression so that the nerves

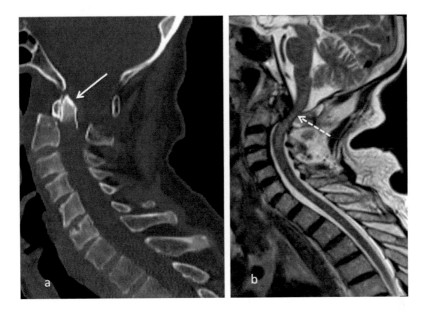

Figure 4.16 Sagittal reformatted CT image (a) and sagittal T2W MR image (b) in a patient with posteriorly displaced fracture of the dens. The MR image clearly shows the extent of cord compression by the displaced fracture fragment (*dashed white arrow, b*).

stand out brightly against a dark background. It is the best imaging modality to evaluate peripheral neuropathies.

Q3. What is SCIWORA and in whom is it commonly seen?
Answer: SCIWORA is spinal cord injury without radiographic abnormality. It is more commonly seen in children younger than 8 years of age due to larger head size, weak neck muscles and increased elasticity of vertebral ligaments.

CASE-BASED REVIEWS

Cervical spine trauma

CASE HISTORY

A 60-year-old man presented with paraparesis following a road traffic accident. There was injury in the cervical spine region. An MRI was done to understand the extent and severity of injury to plan further management.

IMAGING FINDINGS

MRI of the cervical spine showed the following findings (Figure 4.17a, b):

- Hemorrhagic cord contusion extending from C2 to D4 level with altered cord signal and intraparenchymal hemorrhage

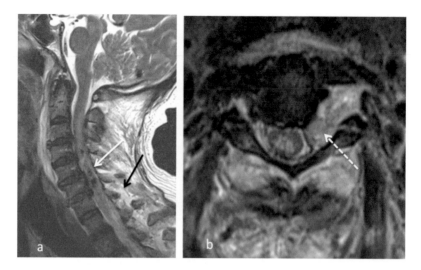

Figure 4.17 Sagittal T2W image (a) showing hemorrhagic cord contusion (*white arrow*), fracture of the spinous processes (*black arrow*) and axial T2W image (b) showing hemorrhagic pseudomeningocoele in the left C3/4 neural foramen (*dashed white arrow*).

- Hemmorhagic pseudomeningocele on the left at C3/4 level, suggestive of pre-ganglionic avulsion injury to the left C4 nerve root
- Fracture of the spinous processes of multiple cervical and dorsal vertebrae with extensive surrounding soft tissue edema
- Prevertebral soft tissue edema
- Spondylotic changes and multilevel degenerative disc disease

DISCUSSION

A significant number of patients with road traffic accidents have injury to the cervical spine. Prompt diagnosis is important as missed or delayed diagnosis of cervical spine injury can lead to a permanent neurological deficit.

There are different mechanisms of injury involving the cervical spine, which include flexion injuries, extension injuries and axial compression injuries.

Q1. What determines the prognosis of a patient with cervical spine injury?
Answer. The prognosis depends upon:
- The mechanism of injury
- Whether the injury is stable or unstable
- Presence and nature of cord contusion

Q2. Which injuries are considered unstable?
Answer. Unstable injuries include:
- Bilateral interfacetal dislocation
- Flexion/extension teardrop fracture

- Wedge fracture with posterior ligamentous rupture
- Burst fractures

Q3. What are the types of cord contusions seen on MRI?
Answer. Spinal cord contusions are of two types:
- Non-hemorrhagic contusion, when there is only cord oedema
- Hemorrhagic parenchymal contusion with T2 low signal intensity within the oedema

The length of the cervical spinal cord involved and the nature of contusion are factors which influence the prognosis. Hemorrhagic contusion indicates poorer prognosis.

Nerve injury due to prolonged ICU stay

CASE HISTORY

A 38-year-old man presented with history of gradual-onset weakness of the right upper limb. He has a history of a prolonged course of hospitalization and ICU admission for COVID-19 illness 2 months prior, requiring intubation and prone positioning

On clinical examination, there was suspicion of right-sided brachial plexopathy. There was no history of trauma or fever in the interim period. The routine blood investigations including CBC, CRP and ESR were within normal limits.

IMAGING FINDINGS

MRI of the cervical spine was done, which showed mild cervical disc bulges without significant spinal cord or nerve root compression to explain the right upper limb weakness (Figure 4.18a). EMG/NCV suggested upper-trunk brachial plexopathy with axonal degeneration. The exact site, severity and nature of the nerve involvement could not be delineated.

An MRI of the brachial plexus with neurography was then done to answer the stated concerns. The brachial plexus MRI showed mild diffuse edema of the right supraspinatus and infraspinatus muscles (Figure 4.18b). This was consistent with denervation edema. The MR neurography showed mild thickening with increased signal in the right suprascapular nerve (Figure 4.18c). The nerve continuity was maintained. There was no extrinsic mass/haematoma causing compression of the nerve. There were no signs of inflammation in the surrounding soft tissues.

Imaging findings and correlation with clinical features and electrophysiological tests favour a positioning-related injury (axonotmesis) of the suprascapular nerve.

DISCUSSION

Peripheral nerve imaging by both high-resolution USG and MRI with MR neurography has a very important role in the diagnosis and management of patients with suspected nerve pathologies. Such pathologies are being increasingly seen in

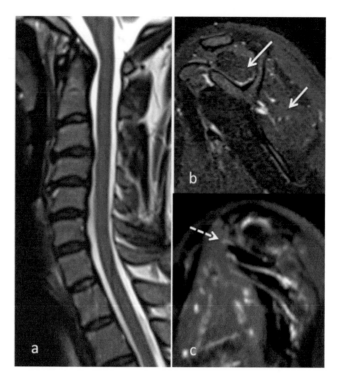

Figure 4.18 Sagittal T2W image of the cervical spine (a) showing mild disc bulges without cord compression and sagittal STIR image of rotator cuff muscles (b) showing mild edema in the right supraspinatus and infraspinatus muscles (*white arrows*). Reconstructed 3D STIR MIP sagittal image (c) showing mild thickening of the right suprascapular nerve with hyperintense signal (*white dashed arrow*).

patients with coronavirus disease, both during the disease course and also after recovery, as a complication of treatment and prolonged hospitalization course.

Q1. What are the causes of peripheral nerve involvement in patients with COVID-19?

Answer. Causes of peripheral nerve involvement in COVID-19 patients are:

- Post-infectious inflammatory neuropathy
- Systemic neuropathy
- Nerve entrapment secondary to hematoma
- Prone positioning–related injury

Q2. What are the advantages and limitations of high-resolution USG for imaging of peripheral nerves?

Answer. The advantages of USG include:

- Cost effective
- Widely available
- High spatial resolution

- Dynamic scanning
- Comparison with the contralateral side

The limitations of USG include:

- Operator dependence
- Inability to adequately assess deep-seated nerves or those subjacent to osseous structures
- Limited utility in the presence of scarring

Q3. What are the advantages and limitations of MRI for imaging of peripheral nerves?

Answer. The advantages of MRI include:
- High contrast resolution
- Multiplanar imaging
- Can assess deep-seated nerves
- Simultaneously assess adjacent osseous and soft tissue structures
- Denervation changes in muscles

The limitations of MRI include:

- High cost
- Limited availability
- Long scan time
- Contraindicated in patients with pacemakers and cochlear implants
- Cannot be done in patients with severe claustrophobia

ACKNOWLEDGMENTS

The authors would like to acknowledge Dr Narayanam Anantha Sai Kiran, Associate Professor, Neurosurgery Department, Narayana Medical College and Hospital, Nellore, who contributed Figures 4.13, 4.14 and 4.15 in the book.

FURTHER READING

1. Hayeri MR, Ziai P, Shehata ML, Teytelboym OM, Huang BK. Soft-tissue infections and their imaging mimics: From cellulitis to necrotizing fasciitis. *Radiographics.* 2016;36(6):1888–910.
2. Lu CH, Tsang YM, Yu CW, Wu MZ, Hsu CY, Shih TT. Rhabdomyolysis: Magnetic resonance imaging and computed tomography findings. *J Comput Assist Tomogr.* 2007;31(3):368–74.
3. Khan FY. Rhabdomyolysis: A review of the literature. *Neth J Med.* 2009;67(9):272–83.
4. Schulze M, Kotter I, Ernemann U, Fenchel M, Tzaribatchev N, Claussen CD, et al. MRI findings in inflammatory muscle diseases and their noninflammatory mimics. *AJR Am J Roentgenol.* 2009;192:1708–16.
5. Pilania K, Jankharia B. Role of MRI in idiopathic inflammatory myopathies: A review article. *Acta Radiol.* 2021 Feb 7:284185121990305, doi: 10.1177/0284185121990305. Epub ahead of print. PMID: 33554607.

6. Ramani SL, Samet J, Franz CK, Hsieh C, Nguyen CV, Horbinski C, et al. Musculoskeletal involvement of COVID-19: Review of imaging. *Skeletal Radiol.* 2021;50(9): 1763–73.

7. Upadhyaya V, Choudur HN. Imaging in peripheral neuropathy: Ultrasound and MRI. *Indian J Musculoskelet Radiol.* 2021;3(1):14–23.

8. Fernandez CE, Franz CK, Ko JH, Walter JM, Koralnik IJ, Ahlawat S, et al. Imaging review of peripheral nerve injuries in patients with COVID-19. *Radiology.* 2021;298(3):E117–E30.

9. Gaskin CM, Helms CA. Parsonage-turner syndrome: MR imaging findings and clinical information of 27 patients. *Radiology.* 2006;240(2):501–7.

10. Scalf RE, Wenger DE, Frick MA, Mandrekar JN, Adkins MC. MRI Findings of 26 patients with parsonage-turner syndrome. *AJR Am J Roentgenol.* 2007;189(1):W39–W44.

11. Upadhyaya V, Upadhyaya DN, Bansal R, Pandey T, Pandey AK. MR neurography in parsonage-turner syndrome. *Indian J Radiol Imaging.* 2019;29(3):264–70.

12. Chandra J, Sheerin F, Lopez de Heredia L, Meagher T, King D, Belci M, et al. MRI in acute and subacute post-traumatic spinal cord injury: Pictorial review. *Spinal Cord.* 2012;50:2–7.

13. Alkan O, Yildirim T, Tokmak N, Tan M. Spinal MRI findings of Guillain-Barre syndrome. *J Radiol Case Rep.* 2009;3(3):25–8.

14. Goh C, Desmond PM, Phal PM. MRI in transverse myelitis. *J Magn Reson Imaging.* 2014;40(6):1267–79.

15. Pierce JL, Donahue JH, Nacey NC, Quirk CR, Perry MT, Faulconer N, et al. Spinal hematomas: What a radiologist needs to know. *Radiographics.* 2018;38(5):1516–35.

16. Hoffman JR, Mower WR, Wolfson AB, Todd KH, Zucker MI. National emergency X-radiography utilization study group. Validity of a set of clinical criteria to rule out injury to the cervical spine in patients with blunt trauma. *N Engl J Med.* 2000;343:94–9.

17. Stiell IG, Clement CM, McKnight RD, Brison R, Schull MJ, Rowe BH, et al. The Canadian C-spine rule versus the NEXUS low-risk criteria in patients with trauma. *N Engl J Med.* 2003;349:2510–18.

18. Harris Jr JH, Carson GC, Wagner LK. Radiologic diagnosis of traumatic occipitovertebral dissociation: 1. Normal occipitovertebral relationships on lateral radiographs of supine subjects. *AJR Am J Roentgenol.* 1994;162(4):881–6.

19. Hoffman JR, Wolfson AB, Todd KH, Mower WR. Selective cervical spine radiography in blunt trauma: Methodology of the national emergency X-radiography utilization study (NEXUS). *Ann Emerg Med.* 1998;32(4):461–9.

20. Harris Jr JH, Carson GC, Wagner LK, Kerr N. Radiologic diagnosis of traumatic occipitovertebral dissociation: 2. Comparison of three methods of detecting occipitovertebral relationships on lateral radiographs of supine subjects. *AJR Am J Roentgenol.* 1994;162(4):887–92.

21. Berritto D, Pinto A, Michelin P, Demondion X, Badr S. Trauma imaging of the acute cervical spine. *Semin Musculoskelet Radiol.* 2017;21(03):184–98.

22. Guarnieri G, Izzo R, Muto M. The role of emergency radiology in spinal trauma. *Br J Radiol.* 2016;89(1061):20150833, doi: 10.1259/bjr.20150833. Epub 2016 Jan 11.

23. Hoffman JR, Schriger DL, Mower W, Luo JS, Zucker M. Low-risk criteria for cervical-spine radiography in blunt trauma: A prospective study. *Ann Emerg Med.* 1992; 21(12):1454–60.

24. Stiell IG, Wells GA, Vandemheen KL, Clement CM, Lesiuk H, Maio VJD, et al. The Canadian C-spine rule for radiography in alert and stable trauma patients. *JAMA.* 2001;286(15):1841–8.

25. Goldberg W, Mueller C, Panacek E, Tigges S, Hoffman JR, Mower WR, NEXUS Group. Distribution and patterns of blunt traumatic cervical spine injury. *Ann Emerg Med.* 2001;38(1):17–21.

26. Lenehan B, Boran S, Street J, Higgins T, McCormack D, Poynton AR. Demographics of acute admissions to a national spinal injuries unit. *Eur Spine J.* 2009;18(7):938–42.

27. Greenbaum J, Walters N, Levy PD. An evidenced-based approach to radiographic assessment of cervical spine injuries in the emergency department. *J Emerg Med.* 2009;36(1):64–71.

28. Varma A, Hill EG, Nicholas J, Selassie A. Predictors of early mortality after traumatic spinal cord injury: A population-based study. *Spine.* 2010;35(7):778–83.

29. Daffner RH, Hackney DB. ACR Appropriateness Criteria on suspected spine trauma. *J Am Coll Radiol.* 2007;4(11):762–75.

30. Bailitz J, Starr F, Beecroft M, Bankoff J, Roberts R, Bokhari F, et al. CT should replace three-view radiographs as the initial screening test in patients at high, moderate, and low risk for blunt cervical spine injury: A prospective comparison. *J Trauma.* 2009;66(6):1605–9.

31. Daffner RH. Cervical radiography for trauma patients: A time-effective technique? *AJR Am J Roentgenol.* 2000;175(5):1309–11.

32. Ryken TC, Hadley MN, Walters BC, Aarabi B, Dhall SS, Gelb DE, et al. Radiographic assessment. *Neurosurgery.* 2013;(72 Suppl 2):54–72.

33. Garrett M, Consiglieri G, Kakarla UK, Chang SW, Dickman CA. Occipitoatlantal dislocation. *Neurosurgery.* 2010;66(3 Suppl):48–55.

34. Karam YR, Traynelis VC. Occipital condyle fractures. *Neurosurgery.* 2010;66(3 Suppl):56–9.

35. Harris Jr JH, Carson GC, Wagner LK. Radiologic diagnosis of traumatic occipitovertebral dissociation: 1. Normal occipitovertebral relationships on lateral radiographs of supine subjects. *AJR Am J Roentgenol.* 1994;162(4):881–6.

36. Harris Jr JH, Carson GC, Wagner LK, Kerr N. Radiologic diagnosis of traumatic occipitovertebral dissociation: 2. Comparison of three methods of detecting occipitovertebral relationships on lateral radiographs of supine subjects. *AJR Am J Roentgenol.* 1994;162(4):887–92.

37. Horn EM, Feiz-Erfan I, Lekovic GP, Dickman CA, Sonntag VK, Theodore N. Survivors of occipitoatlantal dislocation injuries: Imaging and clinical correlates. *J Neurosurg Spine.* 2007;6(2):113–20.

38. Theodore N, Aarabi B, Dhall SS, Gelb DE, Hurlbert RJ, Rozzelle CJ, et al. The diagnosis and management of traumatic atlanto-occipital dislocation injuries. *Neurosurgery.* 2013;(72 Suppl 2):114–26.

39. Wilson J, Harrop J. Update on upper cervical spine injury classifications. *Semin Spine Surg.* 2017;29(1):9–13.

39. Jackson RS, Banit DM, Rhyne III AL, Darden II BV. Upper cervical spine injuries. *J Am Acad Orthop Surg.* 2002;10(4):271–80.

41. Vaccaro AR, Hulbert RJ, Patel AA, Fisher C, Dvorak M, Lehman Jr RA, et al, Spine Trauma study group. The subaxial cervical spine injury classification system: A novel approach to recognize the importance of morphology, neurology, and integrity of the disco-ligamentous complex. *Spine.* 2007;32(21):2365–74.

42. Aarabi B, Walters BC, Dhall SS, Gelb DE, Hurlbert RJ, Rozzelle, et al. Subaxial cervical spine injury classification systems. *Neurosurgery.* 2013;(72 Suppl 2):170–86.

43. Korres D, Benetos IS, Evangelopoulos DS, Athanassacopoulos M. Tear-drop fractures of the lower cervical spine: Classification and analysis of 54 cases. *Eur J Orthop Surg Traumatol.* 2007;17(6):521–6.

44. Anderson SE, Boesch C, Zimmermann H, Busato A, Hodler J, Bingisser R, et al. Are there cervical spine findings at MR imaging that are specific to acute symptomatic whiplash injury? A prospective controlled study with four experienced blinded readers. *Radiology.* 2012;262(2):567–75.

45. Palmieri F, Cassar-Pullicino VN, Dell'Atti C, Lalam RK, Tins BJ, Tyrrell PNM, et al. Uncovertebral joint injury in cervical facet dislocation: The headphones sign. *Eur Radiol.* 2006;16(6):1312–15.

46. Szwedowski D, Walecki J. Spinal cord injury without radiographic abnormality (SCIWORA)- clinical and radiological aspects. *Pol J Radiol.* 2014;79:461–4.

5

Urogenital system

SURABHI VYAS, SMITA MANCHANDA
AND ANIRBAN HOM CHOUDHURI

INTRODUCTION

Many imaging techniques can be performed to evaluate the diseases of the urogenital system. X-rays are not much helpful except sometimes in detecting calculus and monitoring their size and position. USG is good for assessment of swellings and masses in the pelvic region besides the calculi, and can determine the obstructions in different parts of the urogenital tract. They can also guide during biopsies. USG is advantageous in that it is less costly and free from radiation hazards while both plain CT scan and CT angiography carry the risk of radiation exposure. CT angiography carries the additional risk of allergic reaction and contrast-induced kidney injury. MRI provides more detailed information than CT except in urinary calculi. They also provide information about the blood vessels. Besides these modalities, radionuclide scanning can assess kidney blood flow and urine formation. Retrograde urography can diagnose scarring, tumours and fistulas; cystography and cystourethrography are performed to rule out bladder injury and detect valve patency; while angiography can detect vascular abnormalities (Figures 5.1 and 5.2).

AIM OF IMAGING

The aim of imaging in the ICU includes:

- Detecting infective focus in a febrile patient
- Finding the cause of abdominal distension, reduced urinary output and for differentiating obstructive from non-obstructive pathology
- To guide aspiration and drainage
- To evaluate the extent and severity of abdominal and pelvic trauma

DOI: 10.1201/9781003218739-5

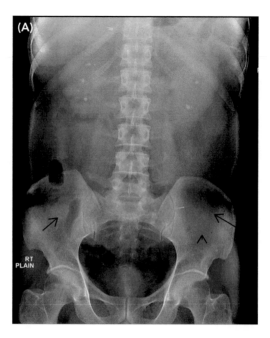

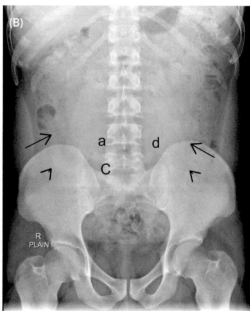

Figure 5.1 Renal and ureteric calculi. Plain radiograph (A) shows multiple radio densities in both lumbar areas (*arrows*) within the renal outlines (*arrowheads*). Plain and prone post-contrast injection images of IVP study (B, C). Axial and coronal CT images show contracted thick-walled renal pelvis (*arrow*, a, d) with hydronephrosis. The left ureter also shows wall thickening and narrowing (C). No excretion of contrast seen from the left kidney on delayed images (B, C).

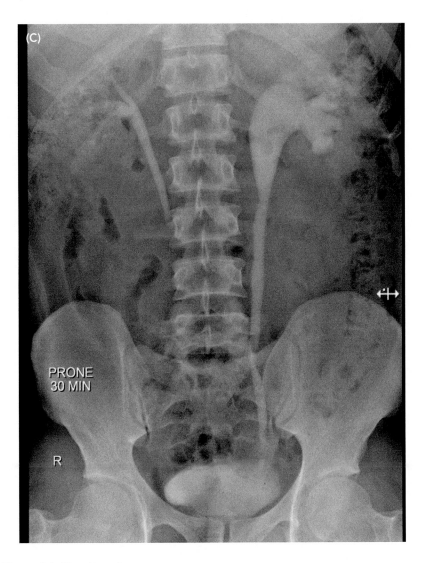

Figure 5.1 (Continued).

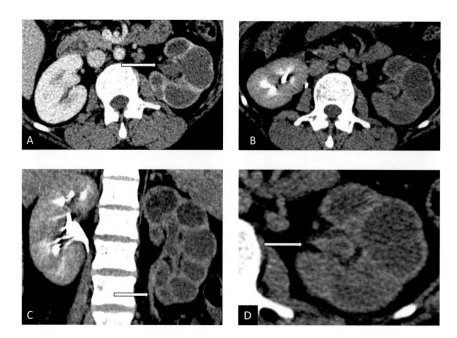

Figure 5.2 Renal and ureteric tuberculosis. Axial and coronal CT images show contracted thick-walled renal pelvis (*arrow*, A, D) with hydronephrosis. The left ureter also shows wall thickening and narrowing (C). No excretion of contrast seen from the left kidney on delayed images (B, C).

IMAGING MODALITIES

A 30-year-old male is admitted following pelvic trauma after a fall with abdominal distension and anuria. He has tachycardia, hypotension and normal sensorium. The abdominal examination suggests ascites with suprapubic tenderness. What are the possible investigations to rule out visceral injury?

The imaging modalities commonly performed in the ICU are X-ray and ultrasonography (USG) as they are usually available bedside and avoid any patient transfer. Computed tomography (CT) is performed to rule out hematoma, detect mass lesion and other findings that cannot be reliably inferred in the USG. MRI can detect finer injuries which can be missed in the CT but is not helpful for calculus.

Bedside imaging

X-ray
- Preferred modality for initial screening and guiding evaluation.
- Supine abdominal radiograph is the most commonly performed.

- Left lateral decubitus AP radiograph or supine cross-table view may be used to detect air-fluid levels and assess free intra-abdominal air.
- Common indications are for detection of calculi and presence of air in the abdominal organs viz. emphysematous pyelonephritis.
- Other indications include confirmation of optimal position of various drainage catheters, tubes and stents.

Ultrasonography (USG)
- Common indications: detection of cause of urinary obstruction, calculi in the urinary system, pyelonephritis, ascites and/or hemoperitoneum.
- Advantages: real-time investigation, wide availability and convenience. Small amounts of fluid may be detected and aspirated.
- Disadvantages: patient habitus, presence of intraperitoneal or air within renal parenchyma, bladder and bowel which may hamper assessment.

Doppler USG
- Doppler can be used as an initial tool for diagnosis of vascular abnormalities viz. renal artery or venous thrombosis, renal artery aneurysm and infarction. It demonstrates either no color flow in the affected vascular segment or dilation of the segment with aberrant flow.
- The examination is challenging in ICU due to poor breath holding by the patient during the procedure, presence of bowel gases and improper patient positioning. Confirmation by CT may be necessary.

Non-bedside imaging

Intravenous pyelography (IVP)
- IVP is rare nowadays as CT urography provides the required information in less time along with a detailed extraluminal evaluation of the urogenital tract.
- IVP demonstrates changes of urinary obstruction in the form of hydronephrosis, hydroureter, ureteric stricture, ureterocele and calculi (Figure 5.1).
- It is the gold standard investigation to demonstrate classical findings of renal tuberculosis such as papillary necrosis, caliceal dilation and infundibular strictures.
- It has a limited role in intensive care practice.

CT
- Non-contrast CT is the modality of choice for evaluation of urinary calculi. CT demonstrates tiny non-obstructing calculi in the urinary tract, which are not detected on USG.
  Dual-energy CT (DECT) provides material composition of the renal calculi.
- CT reveals renal cysts, masses and infections viz. pyeloureteritis, abscess (Figure 5.2).
- CT can assess end-stage renal masses.

- Contrast administration during CT requires normal renal function. Otherwise (eGFR < 30 mL/min/m^2), the risk of acute kidney injury (AKI) due to contrast administration increases as the GFR decreases. This should be kept in mind in the ICU.
- Contrast-enhanced CT (CECT) versus angiography: CECT abdomen is performed in the venous phase unless specific timing of contrast is required for specific organs, for example, triple-phase CT for hepatic mass, CT urography for renal evaluation etc. Angiography study is performed to demonstrate the opacified arterial system, and this requires specific timing for contrast administration.

MRI

- MRI is indicated in renal vascular thrombosis, characterizing renal masses, differentiation of cystic from solid lesions (ultrasound is also used to differentiate cystic from solid masses) and in cases where contrast CT is contraindicated either due to renal compromise or pregnancy.
- Contrast-enhanced MRI is also indicated in suspected prostatic carcinoma.
- MRI contrast and pregnancy: use of contrast is contraindicated in pregnancy as the contrast can cross the placenta, but it can be used when benefits outweigh the fetal risk.
- MRI contrast and renal compromise: in diminished renal function due to chronic kidney disease, the risk of nephrogenic systemic fibrosis (NSF) is common with group 1 gadolinium-based contrast agents (GBCA) and least with group 2 GBCA.

EVALUATION OF FLUID AND HEMOPERITONEUM

A 25-year-old female presents in her 30th week of pregnancy with bleeding p/v, abdominal pain and respiratory distress after a fall. She is pale with tachycardia and hypotension. What are the useful modalities of investigation in the initial phase?

Ascites and hemoperitoneum

- **FAST**
    - Ultrasound abdomen in trauma patients is done as a part of FAST (focused assessment with sonography for trauma) examination.
    - It provides estimation of fluid in the peritoneal cavity. The same may be employed for evaluation of free intraperitoneal fluid in non-traumatic patients and in those with shock and hypotension, where it is part of the RUSH (rapid ultrasound for shock and hypotension) protocol.

- The protocol requires 150–200 mL of fluid in the peritoneal cavity to be detectable on USG.
- It is a B-mode, real-time USG evaluation using a curvilinear 2–5MHz probe, with the patient in supine position.
- USG at right upper quadrant for the hepatorenal recess, right paracolic gutter, right sub-diaphragmatic area, left upper quadrant for splenorenal recess, sub-diaphragmatic area and left paracolic gutter and the suprapubic scan for free fluid in the pelvis (recto-vesical, recto-uterine and vesico-uterine pouches) are the sites for assessment of intraperitoneal fluid. In addition, the sub-xiphoid view is used for pericardial fluid diagnosis.
- Pelvis, paracolic spaces and hepatorenal pouch are the sites for detecting small amounts of fluid.
- USG has limited value in diagnosing the source of bleed in the case of hemoperitoneum. It may reveal other causes of fluid accumulation in peritoneal cavity such as renal or hepatic abnormalities or gynaecological complication.

SPECIFIC DISEASES

A 50-year-old male patient undergoes PCNL after recurrent nephrolithiasis. After 10 days of discharge, he presents with high-grade fever, dysuria and mild haematuria. What are the useful investigation modalities in this patient?

Obstructive uropathy

- Ultrasound is valuable as a renal screening modality for obstruction caused by calculus disease and other causes such as pyonephrosis (Figure 5.3).

Pyelonephritis

- Pyelonephritis is inflammation of both the renal pelvis and the renal parenchyma and may be accompanied by obstructive and non-obstructive features.
- Bacterial infections, granulomatous diseases and metabolic diseases can cause pyelonephritis.
- The patient usually presents with pain, fever and urinary burning sensation.
- USG helps to diagnose antecedent abnormalities such as renal calculus disease, renal cysts and abscesses.
- USG may be normal in early interstitial nephritis, or else may show renal enlargement and altered echogenicity (appearing as hypoechoic due to oedema or as hyperechoic due to haemorrhage). It may reveal ill-defined, wedge-shaped hypoechoic areas in the renal parenchyma.

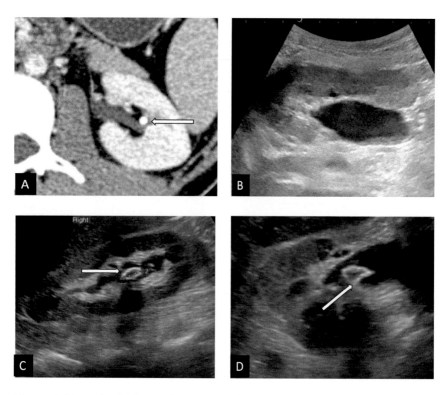

Figure 5.3 Renal calculi. Axial CECT (A) shows a small non-obstructing hyper-dense focus in the left caliceal system (*arrow*). Transverse USG image (B) shows mildly dilated renal pelvis due to distal calculus. Longitudinal (C) and transverse (D) USG image show a calculus in the renal pelvis (*arrow*) with mild hydronephrosis.

- CT has higher sensitivity in diagnosing pyelonephritis and shows areas of differential enhancement with striated nephrogram in the nephrographic phase. Wedge-shaped hypodense areas can be seen in the delayed phases (Figure 5.4). Thickening and enhancement of the urothelial lining can also be seen, along with stranding and inflammatory changes in the surrounding fat (Figure 5.5a, b).
- Complications of acute pyelonephritis in the form of abscess formation result in well-defined round to irregular hypoechoic areas within the renal paren-chyma with frequent perinephric fluid extension. CT demonstrates the abscess as hypodense areas with enhancing walls (Figure 5.6). Perinephric collections and surrounding inflammatory changes are more pronounced in the presence of renal abscess and mirror with clinical deterioration.

Pyonephrosis

- Pyonephrosis refers to an infected obstructed and dilated renal collecting system.

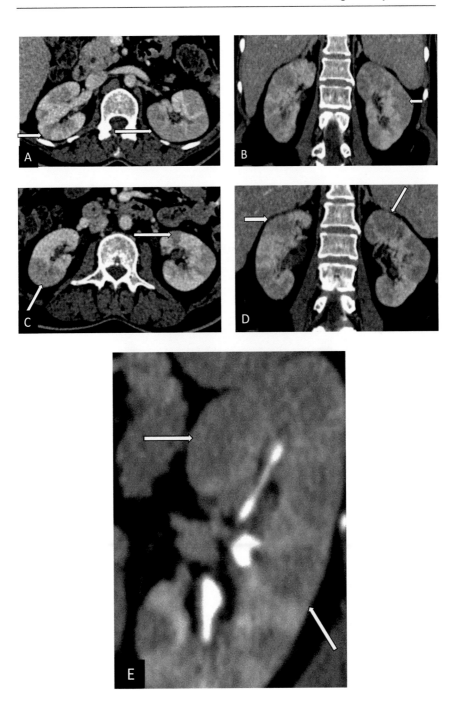

Figure 5.4 Pyelonephritis. Axial and coronal CECT images (A–D) show multiple wedge-shaped areas of differential enhancement in the bilateral renal parenchyma (*arrows*). Similar wedge-shaped areas are seen more clearly in the delayed image (E).

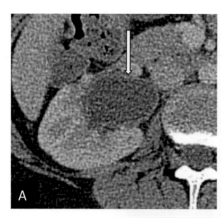
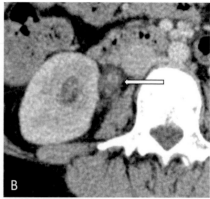
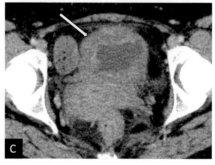

Figure 5.5 Pyelonephritis, ureteritis and cystitis. Axial CECT image (A) shows thickening and enhancement of the urothelium of the renal pelvis, suggestive of pyelonephritis. There is also similar thickening and surrounding fat stranding around the right ureter (B, *arrow*). Axial image of the pelvis (C) shows diffuse thickening and enhancement of the wall of the urinary bladder.

- Patients are usually toxic at presentation, with painful bulging flanks and tenderness.
- USG demonstrates dilated renal pelvicaliceal system with internal echoes (Figure 5.7).
- CT shows thickening of urothelium by more than 2 mm with highly attenuated contents within. Contrast material may accumulate in the dilated collecting system due to stasis. Associated cystitis may also be seen as thickened wall of the urinary bladder with debris or internal echoes (Figure 5.5c).

A 60-year-old post-operative diabetic female after a prolonged ICU stay develops pain during micturition, intermittent low-grade fever, and pain and tenderness of the lower abdomen. Her urine culture is normal, although the routine urine examination shows RBC casts. What are the useful radiological investigations?

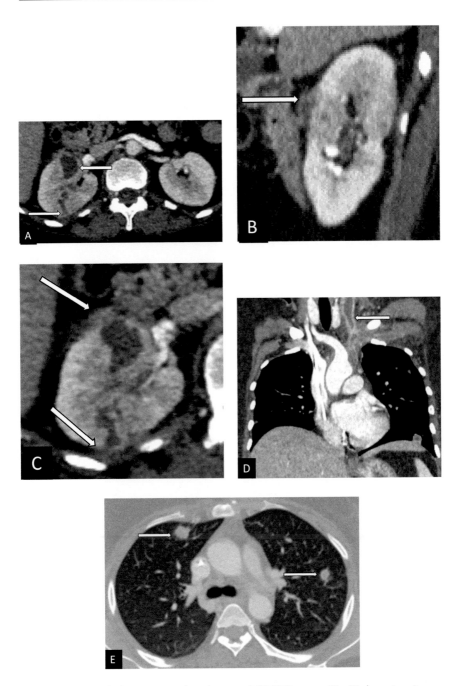

Figure 5.6 Renal abscess. Axial and coronal CECT images (A–C) show two irregular hypodense lesions in the right renal parenchyma with thin enhancing walls
suggestive of abscesses (*arrows*). Perinephric extension of collections are also
seen (*arrow*, C). Left jugular and brachiocephalic vein thrombus are seen (*arrow*,
D), with multiple septic emboli in the lungs (E).

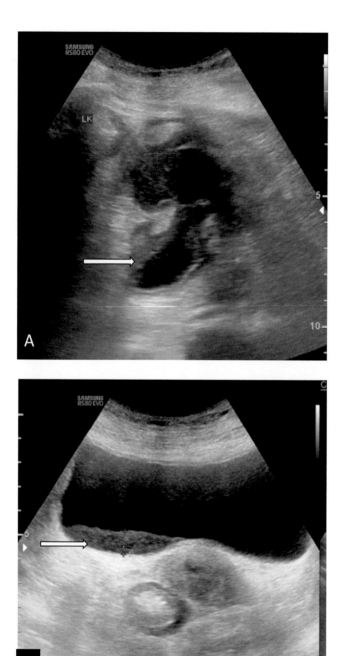

Figure 5.7 Pyonephrosis. Transverse image of the kidney shows thickened urothelium and low-level internal echoes within the pelvicalaceal system (A). Layering of debris is also seen in the urinary bladder (*arrow*, B).

Emphysematous pyelonephritis

- Emphysematous pyelonephritis is a potentially life-threatening infection of the kidneys with gas-forming organisms.
- It is associated with poorly controlled diabetes mellitus in the majority of affected patients.
- USG may demonstrate extensive shadowing and mottling due to the air within the renal parenchyma. CT has greater sensitivity to demonstrate both the presence and extent of disease.
- CT can also differentiate emphysematous pyelitis from emphysematous pyelonephritis by demonstrating air within the renal parenchyma, as opposed to the former, in which air is confined to the collecting system (Figure 5.8).

Acute renal injury

- Ultrasound is the initial modality of evaluation in a case of acute kidney injury (AKI).
- The size, shape and echogenicity of the kidney along with dilatation of the collecting system gives valuable information regarding the cause of AKI.
- CT and MRI are helpful in identifying the cause of injury and demonstrating other features.

Renal hypoperfusion and dysfunction

- Doppler ultrasound is used as a marker for renal dysfunction and hypoperfusion.
- Renal Doppler RI (resistive index) of more than 0.7 is considered abnormal and associated with shock.
- Global renal perfusion on color Doppler also correlates with acute kidney injury and can be easily performed in the intensive care setting using a curvilinear probe.

TUBES AND CATHETERS

Percutaneous Nephrostomy (PCN)

- PCN is indicated for relieving a urinary system obstruction, infection or as a diversion.
- It can also be used as a conduit for treatment of calculus disease.
- PCN is a SIR class 3 procedure.
- It can be performed under ultrasound and/or fluoroscopic guidance.
- A dilated posterior calyx is the preferred site for placement of nephrostomy catheter.

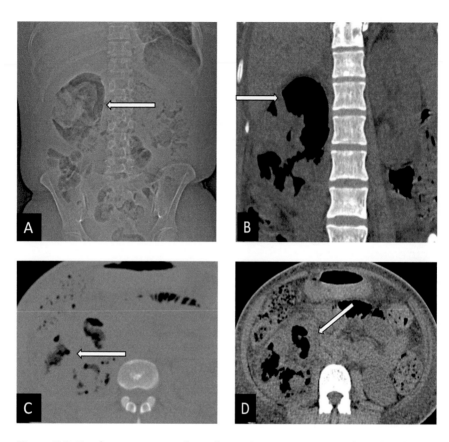

Figure 5.8 Emphysematous pyelonephritis. Scout image (A) and axial and coronal CT images (B–D) show presence of air within the enlarged heterogeneous right kidney. Mottled contents and fluid collection are also seen on the lung window settings (C).

Ureteral stent

- Ureteral or ureteric stents are catheters to ensure free drainage of the urine across the ureters from kidneys.
- The stent can be placed anterograde under fluoroscopic guidance or retrograde under cystoscopic guidance.
- The proximal end is positioned in the renal pelvis and distal end is positioned in the urinary bladder (Figure 5.9).

Bladder and urethral catheterization

- Bladder and urethral catheterization under imaging guidance is performed in ICU patients for monitoring of urine output, microbiological and biochemical analysis and relief of bladder outlet obstruction with less procedural risk.

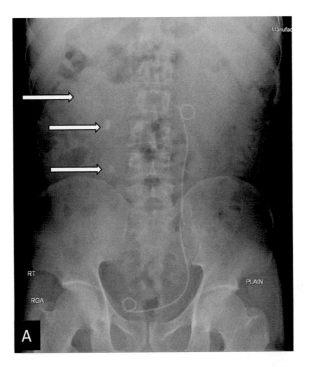

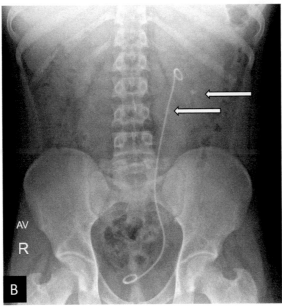

Figure 5.9 Double J stent. Left-sided DJ stent in different cases. Plain radiographs (A, B) show left DJ stent in both cases, with right ureteric and renal calculi in (A) and left renal and ureteric calculi in (B, *arrows*).

- Suprapubic catheters are surgically inserted through the pelvis into the bladder.
- USG demonstrates the position of the catheter tip in the posterior urethra or the bladder lumen in difficult catheterization.
- Difficult catheterization may be facilitated with the aid of USG guidance and trans-rectal pressure measurement.

NORMAL KUB (KIDNEY URETER BLADDER) RADIOGRAPH – READING

- KUB radiograph includes the region extending from the upper pole of kidney superiorly to the inferior pubic rami inferiorly. In contrast, a supine abdominal radiograph also covers the area superior to the diaphragmatic contour.
- Reading of a KUB radiograph should proceed systematically so as not to miss any important and subtle findings.
- The position, size and orientation of the renal shadows is noted first, along with the psoas shadows on either side. The renal shadows extend from L1 to L3 vertebral bodies. The orientation of kidneys is such that the upper poles are directed medially and lower poles are directed laterally.
- Abnormal density within or surrounding the renal shadows are noted for calculi, presence of air or obscuration.
- Presence, number and shape of any renal calculi is noted.
- The psoas shadows on either side of the spine may be obscured in the presence of a renal or para-spinal pathology.
- Calculi along the course of ureters are seen next, followed by the bladder region within the true pelvis.
- The region inferior to the pubic symphysis is noted to ensure that no calculus lies in the course of the urethra.

GYNAECOLOGY

A 70-year-old female with urinary incontinence undergoes pelvic floor repair operation. On the third post-operative day, she develops vaginal bleeding and lower abdominal pain. What are the useful imaging modalities for diagnosis and workup?

KEY INDICATIONS AND IMAGING MODALITIES

- Acute pelvic pain and bleeding per vaginum are a common presentation in the emergency department.
- Imaging along with the clinical findings plays a key role in determining the etiology and distinguish gynecological from gastrointestinal/urological emergencies.

- Ultrasound is the baseline imaging modality. It is fast, highly sensitive, readily available, easy to access and of less cost. The biggest advantage is the portability and ease of bedside evaluation (1).
- CT is often used in the emergency settings, especially when the localization is difficult on the basis of symptoms alone. In addition, CT is required for extent delineation of large abscess/hematomas (2).
- MRI is not usually used in the acute setting and is often used for problem solving in indeterminate USG/CT findings. MRI is beneficial in evaluation of Mullerian anomalies, tumours and endometrial pathologies. This section focuses on the clinical presentation and key imaging features of the common gynaecological emergencies.

COMMON DISEASE ENTITIES

Pelvic inflammatory disease

- This includes a spectrum of diseases such as endometritis, salpingitis, tubo-ovarian complex, pyosalpinx and peritonitis.
- The common etiological agents include *Chlamydia trachomatis*, *Neisseria gonorrhoea*, *Mycoplasma genitalium* and other gram-negative bacteria (3). Usually sexually transmitted, there is spread of infection from the vagina to the other female reproductive organs.
- Varying degrees of pelvic pain with vaginal discharge and cervical excitation are seen on examination. In the initial stages, imaging may be normal. These patients can present with acute pain in the emergency setting. There may be associated thrombophlebitis, which can aggravate to clinical sepsis.
- USG shows uterine enlargement, thickened endometrium, hydrosalpinx/pyosalpinx and tubo-ovarian abscesses, which are the typical sonographic manifestations (Figure 5.10) (4).
- On CT, tubo-ovarian abscesses are seen as complex adnexal masses with thick walls and septations and peripheral enhancement. Parapelvic fat stranding, ascites and thickened uterosacral ligaments are usually identified (Figure 5.11) (5).
- MRI reveals inflammation in the parametrium as ill-defined hyperintense areas on T2FS images. A dilated, fluid-filled, tortuous C- or S-shaped structure with T1 and T2 intermediate signal contents is suggestive of pyosalpinx. Thick-walled, fluid-filled abscesses are seen as heterogeneous T1 and T2 signal intensity (pus, haemorrhage and debris) with peripheral rim enhancement.

Rupture of hemorrhagic cyst/endometriotic cyst

- Corpus luteum rupture is a common cause of acute pelvic pain in women, but the resulting hemoperitoneum in some patients can be potentially life threatening.
- A higher incidence of rupture of corpus luteum is seen in patients with congenital bleeding disorders and those on anticoagulants (2, 6). Rarely, even the endometriotic cysts can rupture.

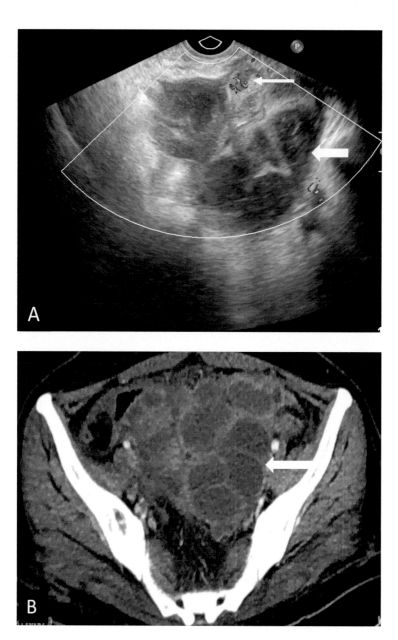

Figure 5.10 Pelvic inflammatory disease in a 32-year-old female with fever, pain in the abdomen and discharge per vaginum. (A) Transvaginal sonogram shows bilateral, thick-walled, complex multilocular cystic lesions with internal echoes (*block arrow*) and mild peripheral vascularity (*arrow*). (B) Axial CECT shows adnexal multilocular cystic masses (*solid arrow*) with thick, enhancing septae, loss of normal ovarian parenchyma and surrounding fat stranding.

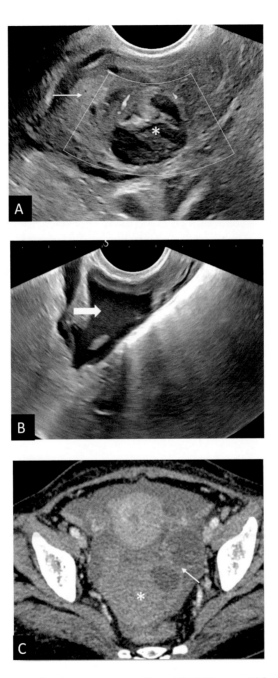

Figure 5.11 Haemorrhagic cyst rupture. (A and B) A 21-year-old female with acute pain in the abdomen on day 16 of menstrual cycle. TVS revealed left ovarian cyst (*) with irregular, crenated margin and internal echogenic contents. Adjacent echogenic hematoma (*arrow*) and free fluid with echogenic debris/hemoperitoneum (*solid arrow*) suggestive of ruptured corpus luteum. (C) Axial CECT image in another patient shows cyst in left ovary (*arrow*) with irregular wall along with hyperdense free fluid in the pelvis (*).

- Patients in the reproductive age group classically present with acute pelvic pain usually in the luteal phase of their cycle. The patient can be hemodynamically unstable if there is a large amount of hemorrhagic ascites. On vaginal examination, there is tenderness along with pain on lifting up the cervix. The haemodynamically stable patients can be managed conservatively as this entity is self-limiting. However, urgent exploration laparotomy is essential for patients who are in shock.
- USG reveals internal echogenic foci within a hemorrhagic cyst, which is thick-walled and with crenulated margins. The cyst shows peripheral vascularity on color Doppler evaluation. USG may also reveal highly echogenic blood clots surrounding the uterus and adnexa. Hemoperitoneum is seen as fluid with echogenic mobile contents/debris (Figure 5.11) (7).
- CT reveals a complex adnexal cystic lesion with thick, irregular, enhancing wall and internal hyperdense contents. Rupture is suggested by a focal discontinuity in the cyst wall. Active contrast extravasation from the cyst confirms the diagnosis but is a rare finding. Hyperdense foci may be seen in the adnexa and are suggestive of a sentinel clot. The presence of high attenuation free fluid is suggestive of hemoperitoneum (Figure 5.11) (6, 7).
- MRI can be used as a problem-solving tool in patients presenting with hemoperitoneum and a suspected gynaecological cause. However, because of limited availability and long scan durations, it is not much used in critical care settings. MRI reveals a well-defined cyst with thick enhancing wall and iso- to hyperintense contents on T1-weighted images (7). Hemoperitoneum can have a variable appearance on T1W and T2W images depending upon the age of bleed.

Tumour rupture

- Rupture of benign mature cystic teratoma or dermoids can perforate into adjacent viscera such as bladder and bowel, necessitating ICU admission. Although less common, malignant tumour can also rupture from increased intralesional pressure (anticoagulant therapy) or pregnancy, leading to bleeding and shock because of hemoperitoneum. There may be associated features of peritonitis. Imaging is very important to aid in diagnosis and management.
- USG may show a change in the size of pre-existing lesion with irregular margins and the presence of echogenic ascites, which suggests tumour rupture.
- CT shows alteration in shape and reduction in size of previous tumour with irregular wall thickening in contrast-enhanced scan. The presence of high-density ascites, sentinel clot sign or fluid-fluid level within lesion suggests tumour rupture. In teratoma, fat deposits may be seen in peritoneum with peritoneal thickening and enhancement (Figure 5.12). In perforation of dermoid cyst into adjacent viscera, fat may be seen within the bladder, or echogenic strands of hair may be visible within the bladder and urethra.

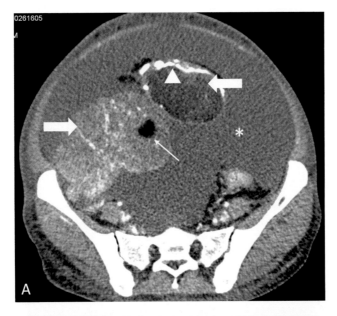

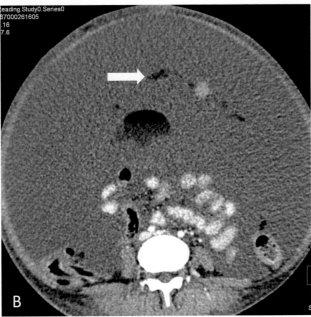

Figure 5.12 Ovarian malignant teratoma with rupture. A 30-year-old female with progressive abdominal distension. (A) Axial CECT image shows bilateral adnexal masses (*solid arrow*) with fat attenuation contents (*arrow*). The left adnexal mass shows rim calcification (*arrowhead*). Gross ascites (*) and peritoneal thickening are seen. (B) In a cranial section, there are soft tissue and fat attenuation deposits (*arrow*).

- MRI can be performed in stable patients. It shows the presence of high signal-intensity ascites or sentinel clot adjacent to the site of rupture. Contained rupture can be seen as a discontinuity in the tumour capsule with an adjacent loculated collection or tumour extension.

CONCLUSION

In the ICU, X-ray and USG are preferred imaging modalities due to their bedside availability, although they have their limitations. When in doubt, cross-sectional imaging (CT, MRI) can delineate disease extent and aid lesion characterization.

FURTHER READING

1. Kaakaji Y, Nghiem HV, Nodell C, Winter TC. Sonography of obstetric and gynecologic emergencies: Part II, gynecologic emergencies. *AJR.* 2000;174:651–6.
2. Roche O, Chavan N, Aquilina J, Rockall A. Radiological appearances of gynaecological emergencies. *Insights Imaging.* 2012;3:265–75.
3. Foti PV, et al. Cross-sectional imaging of acute gynaecologic disorders: CT and MRI findings with differential diagnosis – part II: Uterine emergencies and pelvic inflammatory disease. *Insights Imaging.* 2019;10:118.
4. Bhalla D, Manchanda S, Vyas S. Algorithmic approach to sonography of adnexal masses: An evolving paradigm. *Curr Probl Diagn Radiol.* 2021 Sep–Oct;50(5):703–15, doi: 10.1067/j.cpradiol.2020.08.008. Epub 2020 Aug 26. PMID: 32958313.
5. Aggarwal A, Das CJ, Manchanda S. Imaging spectrum of female genital tuberculosis: A comprehensive review. *Curr Probl Diagn Radiol.* 2021 July 6:S0363–0188(21)00112–2, doi: 10.1067/j.cpradiol.2021.06.014. Epub ahead of print. PMID: 34304946.
6. Tonolini M, et al. Cross-sectional imaging of acute gynaecologic disorders: CT and MRI findings with differential diagnosis – part I: Corpus luteum and haemorrhagic ovarian cysts, genital causes of haemoperitoneum and adnexal torsion. *Insights Imaging.* 2019;10:119.
7. Pulappadi VP, Manchanda S, Sk P, Hari S. Identifying corpus luteum rupture as the culprit for haemoperitoneum. *Br J Radiol.* 2021 Jan 1;94(1117):20200383, doi: 10.1259/bjr.20200383. Epub 2020 Aug 26. PMID: 32822245; PMCID: PMC7774694.
8. American College of Radiology. ACR manual on contrast media v10.3. *Nephrogenic Systemic Fibrosis.* www.acr.org/~/media/ACR/documents/PDF/QualitySafety/resources/contrast-manual/Contrast_Media.
9. Von Kuenssberg Jehle D, Stiller G, Wagner D. Sensitivity in detecting free intraperitoneal fluid with the pelvic views of the FAST exam. *Am J Emerg Med.* 2003 Oct;21(6):476–8.
10. Deoraj S, Zakharious F, Nasim A, et al. Emphysematous pyelonephritis: Outcomes of conservative management and literature review. *Case Reports.* 2018;bcr-2018–225931.
11. Barozzi L, Valentino M, Santoro A, Mancini E, Pavlica P. Renal ultrasonography in critically ill patients. *Crit Care Med.* 2007;35(Suppl):S198–205.
12. Schnell D, Reynaud M, Venot M, Le Maho AL, Dinic M, Baulieu M, et al. Resistive index or color-Doppler semi-quantitative evaluation of renal perfusion by inexperienced physicians: Results of a pilot study. *Minerva Anestesiol.* 2014;80:1273–81.

13. Kameda T, Murata Y, Fujita M, Isaka A. Transabdominal ultrasound-guided urethral catheterization with transrectal pressure. *J Emerg Med.* 2014;46:215–19.
14. Park SB, Kim JK, Kim KR, Cho KS. Imaging findings of complications and unusual manifestations of ovarian teratomas. *Radiographics.* 2008 July–Aug;28(4):969–83, doi: 10.1148/rg.284075069. PMID: 18635624.
15. Salvadori PS, et al. Spontaneous rupture of ovarian cystadenocarcinoma: Pre- and post-rupture computed tomography evaluation. *Radiol Bras.* 2015;48(5):330–3.

6

Gastrointestinal system

ASHISH VERMA, SAKSHI DUGGAL AND ISHAN KUMAR

INTRODUCTION

Abdominal imaging is performed in the ICU to diagnose acute abdomen, evaluate post-operative recovery, assess severity of abdominal sepsis, polytrauma, multiorgan dysfunction, tropical infections, poisoning and many other conditions (Table 6.1 and Table 6.2).

> A 25-year-old patient with blunt trauma of abdomen following accident is brought in with altered sensorium, bleeding with features of shock. After being resuscitated his sensorium improves, blood pressure and heart rate stabilizes, but the patient continues to have abdominal distension and pain. What are the abdominal imaging modalities useful in this patient?

AIM OF IMAGING

a. To look for abdominal fluid collections and to quantify the same
b. To investigate the causes for mechanical or functional bowel obstruction
c. To screen an otherwise unresponsive person for abdominal causes of hemodynamic alteration
d. To evaluate abdominal viscera for suspected dysfunction

> If you are suspecting a splenic rupture, which imaging modalities would you rely upon? Also, if the shock doesn't improve after resuscitation with fluids and inotropes, what additional imaging modalities would be useful to guide therapy?

DOI: 10.1201/9781003218739-6

Table 6.1 Overview of Acute Abdominal Conditions in ICU That Require Abdominal Imaging (listed in order of frequency per organ) (1)

Esophagus	Stomach	Duodenum	Small Intestine	Colon	Liver	Gall Bladder	Pancreas	Spleen	Vascular	Uterus
Boerhaave syndrome	Peptic ulcer perforation	Peptic ulcer perforation	Ischemic bowel	Appendicitis	Blunt and penetrating trauma	Cholecystitis	Acute pancreatitis	Blunt and penetrating trauma	Ruptured abdominal aortic aneurysm (AAA)	Extra uterine pregnancy
Malignancy related perforation	Penetrating trauma	Blunt or penetrating trauma	Incarcerated hernia	Diverticulitis	Acute Liver Failure	Malignancy	Malignancy		Massive rectus sheath haematoma	Pelvic inflammatory disease
Iatrogenic lesion	Malignancy related perforation	Iatrogenic lesion	Penetrating trauma	Ischemic bowel	Acute toxic or ischemic hepatitis	Gallstone perforation	Trauma		Massive retroperitoneal haematoma	Malignancy
Penetrating trauma	Iatrogenic lesion		Inflammatory bowel disease	Inflammatory bowel disease	Iatrogenic lesion	Choledochus cyst (rare)	Iatrogenic lesion			Trauma
			Malignancy related perforation	Malignancy related perforation		Blunt or penetrating trauma				
			Meckel diverticulum	Blunt and penetrating trauma		Iatrogenic lesion				
			Iatrogenic lesion	Iatrogenic lesion						
				Volvulus						

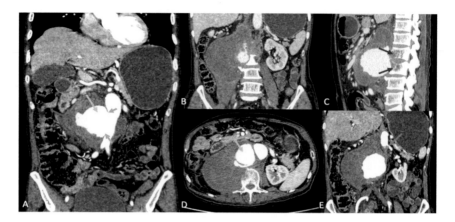

Figure 6.1 Saccular abdominal aortic aneurysm with contained rupture. Axial and multiplanar reconstructed CT aorta angiography show large saccular out-pouching arising from right lateral wall of infrarenal abdominal aorta with wide neck (*green arrow*, A), showing central contrast opacified lumen (*yellow arrow*, A, D), peripheral non-enhancing hypodense thrombus (*blue arrow*, A, D) and throm-bus fissuration (*orange arrow*, B, D). Large retroperitoneal partially thrombosed aneurysm is causing pressure erosion of L2 and L3 vertebral bodies (*red arrow*, C). Circumferential mural thickening of left renal artery ostia causing significant luminal narrowing (*purple arrow*, E).

IMAGING MODALITIES

We shall limit ourselves to the key modalities useful in everyday practice.

Bedside abdominal radiograph

- Best taken in upright (mostly seated) AP position; lateral decubitus views for minimal pleural fluid.
- Quality is usually poor as most mobile radiography systems are not able to give exposure adequate enough for abdomen.
- Not an accurate modality; out of use in most centers now.
- Mostly done to look for calcifications, free air and dilated bowel loops.

Bedside USG

- Investigation of choice for bedside evaluation of abdomen; can be done in any position.
- Done using a combination of low (3–5 Mhz; convex transducer) and high frequency (5–20 Mhz; linear electronic array transducer).
- Mainly used for evaluation of free fluid and dilated bowel loops; careful examination can detect free air as well.
- Simultaneous evaluation of abdomen, thorax and cardiovascular systems may be done.

Table 6.2 Conditions That May Develop during ICU Stay Requiring Abdominal Imaging

Esophagus	Stomach	Small Intestine	Colon	Liver	Gall Bladder	Pancreas
Erosive esophagitis	Stress-related mucosal damage or ulcer; Stomach necrosis or perforation	Stress related mucosal damage or ulcer; Upper GI bleeding	Mucosal damage or ulcer	Toxic or ischemic hepatitis	Atonic bladder	Toxic or ischemic pancreatitis
Bile or acid gastro-esophageal reflux	Upper GI bleeding	Ileus	Lower GI bleeding	Impaired liver synthesis function	Sludge	Asymptomatic biochemical pancreatitis
	Impaired gastric emptying	Mesenteric ischemia	Ileus; Diarrhea; Constipation; Pseudo-obstruction (Ogilvie syndrome); Mesenteric ischemia	Impaired drug metabolism; Ascites	Acalculous cholecystitis	Acute pancreatitis

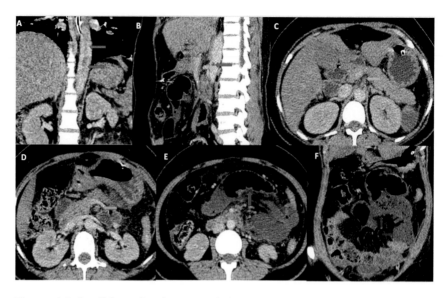

Figure 6.2 Small bowel ischemia with localized perforation in a 45-year-old woman with severe abdominal pain. Axial and multiplanar reconstructed CECT abdomen images show small non-enhancing filling defects in descending thoracic aorta (*pink arrow*, A), abdominal aorta (*blue arrow*, A and B), celiac trunk (*orange arrow*, C) and superior mesenteric artery (*green arrow*, D). Dilated and fluid-filled jejunal loops (*brown arrow*, E) with associated fluid collection in adjacent mesentery and air-fluid levels (*red arrow*, F).

- Can evaluate all type of soft tissue structures including viscera and blood vessels but not bones.
- Can detect the presence of fluid in peritoneal cavity.
- Can differentiate between exudative (slightly echogenic) and transudative (totally anechoic) ascites.
- Can quantify fluid and can ascertain causes of fluid accumulation by virtue of its location.
- Simultaneous evaluation of visceral parenchyma is possible (e.g. presence of chronic liver and kidney disease, liver abscess, hydronephrosis, adrenal hemorrhage, pancreatitis, abdominal lymphadenopathy).
- May be used to guide bedside interventions such as peritoneal tap.
- Can be repeated multiple times as there is no radiation hazard to patient and operator.
- Highly operator dependent, hence expertise is necessary.

CT scan

- Though it is a gold standard investigation in many abdominal conditions, its inability for bedside use is a limiting factor for use in the ICU.

- Accuracy for characterizing the type of effusion is lesser than USG, good to evaluate the cause of ascites/hemoperitoneum in presence of chronic liver and kidney disease, ruptured liver abscess, pancreatitis, unknown malignancy etc.
- Important investigation to determine the cause of abdominal distension or pain that goes undetected on USG (Table 6.3), grading of pancreatitis, detection/staging of malignancies.

In the absence of any definitive findings in USG abdomen, what important information can be gained by performing a CT of the abdomen?

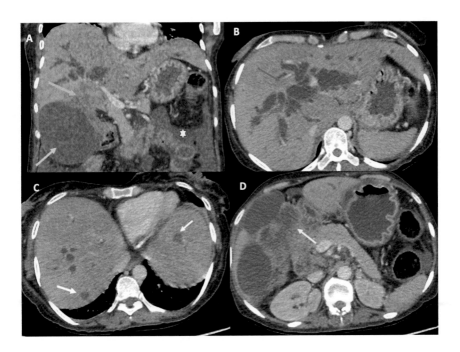

Figure 6.3 Gall bladder neck carcinoma with infiltration of porta hepatis and multiple cholangitic abscess. Image (A) Coronal reformatted CECT shows grossly distended gall bladder (*green arrow*) with a large, ill-defined heterogeneously enhancing multilobulated soft tissue density mass in gall bladder neck region (*yellow arrow*), which is infiltrating adjacent hepatic parenchyma [segment V & IVb], and ascites is also seen (*white star*). Image (B) shows the lesion infiltrating common hepatic duct and biliary confluence at porta hepatis with resultant gross bilobar intrahepatic biliary radical dilatation (*blue arrow*). Images (C and D) axial CECT shows few non-enhancing cystic lesions with heterogenous density in segments II, VII, IVb and V of liver, suggestive of cholangitic abscess (*white arrows*).

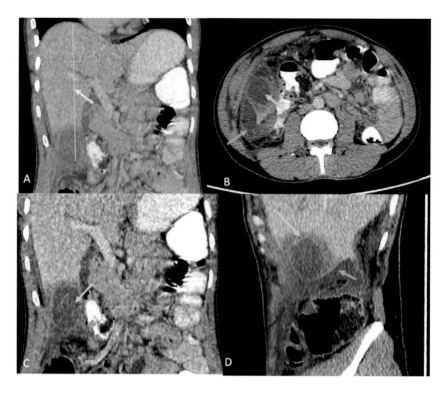

Figure 6.4 Ruptured liver abscess in a 34-year-old male who came with a complaint of right hypochondrium pain. Axial and reformatted CECT images show moderate hepatomegaly (*yellow arrow*, A) with a relatively defined thick-walled peripherally enhancing hypodense lesion (*green arrow*, B, C, D) in segment VI of the liver with associated mild subcapsular fluid collection (*blue arrow*, B, D) communicating with peritoneal cavity (*red arrow*, D).

Table 6.3 Comparative Accuracies of CT Scan and Ultrasonography for Detection of Various Causes of Abdominal Pain

	Sensitivity (%)	Specificity (%)	PPV (%)	NPV (%)
CT scan	36–94	95–100	51–89	96–99
USG	27–76	95–100	30–90	91–99

CARDINAL TECHNICAL POINTERS

- **Peritoneal fluid**: up to 75 mL fluid may be physiological and does not require drainage unless loculation or inflammation is present.
  - *A density of up to 15 HU is considered transudative (high SAAG); density >45 HU indicates presence of blood or high-density material (such as thick pus) in the fluid.*

- **Small bowel obstruction**
  - *For radiography*
    - Use supine position with AP (anteroposterior) projection.
    - As a general rule, the more visible is the small bowel, the more likely is its chance to be pathological.
    - Small bowel is central in location within the abdomen and has characteristic *valvulae conniventes* that traverse the small bowel lumen (haustral folds of colon do not span the entire diameter of the colonic wall).
    - Small bowel loops of diameter more than 3cm are viewed with suspicion. The greater the number of dilated small bowel loops, the more distal is the obstruction.
    - Most underlying causes of small bowel obstruction cannot be diagnosed with an abdominal radiograph.
    - Diagnostic in 50–60% and have high sensitivity only for high-grade obstructions (sensitivity 82%, specificity 84%).
    - A high-grade small bowel obstruction and a low-grade obstruction can be differentiated by the presence of small bowel distention, with maximal dilated loops averaging 36 mm in diameter and exceeding 50% of the caliber of the largest visible colon loop as well as a 2.5 times increase in the number of distended loops in the abdomen compared with the normal number. Other findings are the presence of more than two air-fluid levels, air-fluid levels wider than 2.5 cm, and air-fluid levels differing more than 2 cm in height from one another within the same small bowel loop.
  - *For sonography*
    - Use the supine position, which is not commonly used for the evaluation of SBO mainly because most of the time the bowel loops is filled with gas, producing non-diagnostic sonograms.
    - *Diagnostic features*: dilated fluid-filled small bowel loops with a diameter more than 3 cm, the length of the segment is more than 10 cm, and peristalsis of the dilated segment is increased, as shown by the to-and-fro or whirling motion of the bowel contents.
    - *Cause*: may be determined by examining the area of transition from the dilated to normal bowel.
    - *Severity*: can also be assessed by the presence of free fluid between dilated small bowel loops, aperistalsis and wall thickening (>3 mm) in a fluid-filled distended bowel segment that suggests bowel infarction.

  - *Contrast material–enhanced studies, particularly enteroclysis and CT enteroclysis*: used in clinically suspected low-grade SBO that distends the bowel wall and exaggerates the effects of mild or subclinical obstruction.

  - *Standard CT/MDCT*
    - Sensitivity: 90–96%; Specificity: 96%; Accuracy: 95%
    - Best modality to determine the plan of management.

- CT criteria for small bowel obstruction are the presence of dilated small bowel loops (diameter >2.5 cm from outer wall to outer wall) proximally to normal-caliber or collapsed loops distally.
- Severity: *oral contrast is given* – non-passage of the contrast material beyond the transition point indicates an incomplete bowel obstruction. If *no oral contrast material is given*: presence of high-grade versus incomplete obstruction can be determined by the degree of distal collapse, proximal bowel dilatation, and the presence of the "small bowel feces" sign. Difference in caliber between the proximal dilated bowel and the distal collapsed bowel by more than 50% suggests a high-grade obstruction. Intraluminal particulate material in the proximal dilated segment represents the small bowel feces sign, and it suggests moderate and high-grade obstruction (though controversial).
- Site: the transition point is identified by a change in caliber between the dilated proximal and collapsed distal small bowel loops or by identifying the small bowel feces sign.
- Cause: the answer is almost always in the transition point. Intrinsic bowel lesions manifest as localized mural thickening at the transition point. Extrinsic causes are seen adjacent to the transition point and usually have associated extraintestinal manifestations. Most intraluminal causes manifest as endoluminal "foreign objects" with imaging characteristics different from those of the remaining enteric content.

- **Complications**: strangulation is defined as a closed-loop obstruction associated with intestinal ischemia. Sensitivity of CT is **63–100%**.
- **Diagnostic signs**: thickening and increased attenuation of the affected bowel wall, a halo or "target sign," pneumatosis intestinalis, and gas in the portal vein. A specific finding is lack of wall enhancement; asymmetric enhancement or even delayed enhancement may also be found. Localized fluid and hemorrhage in the mesentery can also be seen.

Large bowel syndrome

Major sites: the cecum, hepatic and splenic flexures, and recto-sigmoid colon. LBO is more common within the left colon.

- **For radiography**

  - *Use supine and nondependent* (either upright or left lateral decubitus) radiographs.
  - Sensitivity: 84%; Specificity: 72%
  - *Normal colonic caliber*: 3 to 8 cm. Dilated caecum > 9 cm, rest of the colon is dilated if > 6 cm.
  - *Diagnostic features*: dilated proximal colon and paucity or absence of gas distal to the obstruction. On the upright or decubitus radiographs, air-fluid levels are often seen in the dilated colon, and their presence suggests

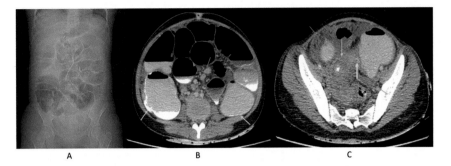

A   B   C

Figure 6.5 Small and large bowel obstruction due to ulcerative colitis: a 14-year-old girl presented with non-passage of flatus and stool. (A) Abdominal radiograph supine AP view shows multiple dilated small and large bowel loops. No free gas is seen, suggesting persistent large bowel obstruction. (B) Axial CECT shows multiple dilated small bowel loops with air-fluid levels, dilated ascending and descending colon (*yellow arrows*) along with multiple enlarged but non-necrotic homogenously enhancing lymph nodes. (C) Axial CECT image shows marked mural thickening (*yellow arrow*) of distal sigmoid colon and marked dilatation of large bowel proximally with transition point marked by *green arrow*. There is no transit of contrast distal to obstruction. Marked perisigmoid and perirectal fat stranding (*blue arrow*) with prominent lymph nodes (*orange arrow*).

acute obstruction as the colonic fluid has not been present long enough to get absorbed.

- **Multidetector CT: diagnostic modality of choice**

  - Sensitivity: 96%; Specificity: 93%
  - *Diagnostic*: dilated large bowel proximal to a transition point and decompressed bowel distal to it. The presence of a transition point is considered a reliable finding for the diagnosis of LBO.

- **Contrast enema: water-soluble iodinated contrast material is used**

  - *Major advantage*: easy distinction between a large bowel obstruction and colonic pseudo-obstruction.
  - *Disadvantage*: for complete evaluation of the colon, the patient must be able to rotate on the fluoroscopy table.

MAJOR CAUSES OF LBO

- *Colon carcinoma*: most common cause, most common locations of obstruction: the sigmoid colon and the splenic flexure. The most common site of perforation is the cecum. CT findings: asymmetric and short-segment colonic wall thickening or an enhancing soft-tissue mass centered in the colon that narrows the colonic lumen with or without findings of ischemia and perforation.
- *Sigmoid volvulus*:

  - *Radiographic signs*: diagnostic in 57–90% of cases. The coffee bean sign/ kidney bean sign or bent inner tube sign (thick 'inner wall' represents the double wall thickness of apposed loops of bowel, with thinner outer walls due to single wall thickness) is seen in both sigmoid volvulus (has few air-fluid levels) and caecal volvulus (has one air-fluid level).

- **Bird beak signs**: seen in all colonic volvuli (describes the smooth, tapering transition point of the obstruction).
  - The **inverted U sign** (an inverted ahaustral dilated sigmoid in the shape of an inverted "U" extending into the right upper quadrant).
    - The **northern exposure sign**: is a high-specificity sign in the sigmoid volvulus [on a supine abdominal radiograph, the apex of the sigmoid volvulus is seen above (cranial to) the transverse colon].
      - The **liver overlap sign**: (the sigmoid loop is seen ascending to the right upper quadrant and projecting over the liver shadow).
- **Absent rectal gas**

  - *CT signs:* all the plain radiographic signs along with **whirl sign** (appearance of spiraled loops of collapsed bowel with enhancing engorged vessels radiating from the twisted bowel at the point of obstruction).
    - *Contrast enema:* water-soluble contrast is used, demonstrates bird beak sign (smooth, tapering transition point of the obstruction).

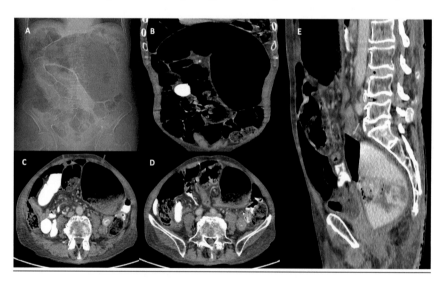

Figure 6.6 Sigmoid volvulus: (A) abdominal radiograph AP view in supine position shows grossly dilated sigmoid colon. (B) CECT coronal reformatted image shows sigmoid colon grossly overdistended with twisting of sigmoid colon, causing resultant closed loop obstruction (coffee bean sign). The ascending and descending loops of the dilated sigmoid colon are conversing on the left side of the pelvis with narrowing of the bowel loops, suggestive of volvulus. The dilated sigmoid is colon reaching up to the left hemidiaphragm. (C, D) Axial CECT: whirl sign (*green arrow*) is noted, representing tension on the tightly twisted mesocolon by the afferent and efferent limbs of the dilated colon. (E) On administration of rectal contrast narrowing/tapering of the sigmoid colon up to the level of obstruction is seen, suggesting bird beak sign (*yellow arrow*).

- Caecal volvulus

  - *Radiography*: diagnostic in 75% cases. Caecal dilatation >9 cm. Caecum rotates out to the left upper quadrant and sometimes into the left lower abdomen or midline.
    - *CT findings*: marked distension of the cecum in an abnormal location, usually in the mid or left upper abdomen; signs of ischemia include wall thickening, mural hypoenhancement, pneumatosis in bowel wall, pneumoperitoneum and/or portal venous gas. Mesenteric stranding and peritoneal fluid help in the diagnosis of bowel wall ischemia. At the site of the twist, a **whirl sign** can be seen.

Acute pancreatitis

> How can we differentiate acute necrotizing from acute interstitial pancreatitis by imaging?

The imaging should be performed 5–7 days after hospital admission when local complications have developed and pancreatic necrosis (if present) should be clearly distinguishable.

Grading
1. *Mild*: discharged within first week, don't require imaging for local complications, but to determine the underlying cause, e.g. gallstones (either USG or MRCP).
2. *Moderately severe*: patients with transient organ failure lasting < 48 hours and/or local or systemic complications.
3. *Severe*: severe disease is characterized by organ failure for > 48 hours.
- *Types*
  1. Interstitial edematous pancreatitis
  2. Necrotizing pancreatitis

- *Radiography*
  - Is insensitive.
  - May demonstrate localized ileus of the small intestine (sentinel loop), spasm of the descending colon (colon cut-off sign).
  - Chest radiographs may demonstrate pleural effusion usually left-sided, hemidiaphragm elevation, basal atelectasis.

- *Ultrasound*
  - Increased pancreatic volume with a marked decrease in echogenicity.
  - Pancreatic body > 2.4 cm in diameter, with marked anterior bowing and surface irregularity.
  - The main role of ultrasound is to look for gallstones, identify areas of necrosis that appear hypoechoic, any thrombosis and collection (parenchymal and peripancreatic).

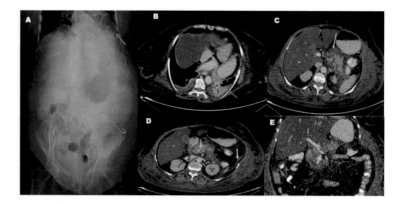

Figure 6.7 Acute necrotizing pancreatitis: scout (A) supine anteroposterior view of abdomen shows gastric shadow and few bowel loops; costophrenic angles appear obliterated (*blue arrow*), suggesting pleural effusion as confirmed on axial CT image (B). (C) Bulky pancreas with fuzzy lobulated border and variable contrast enhancement, there is associated fat stranding (*green arrow*), thickening of left anterior renal, lateroconal fascia (*green arrow*, D) and peripancreatic collection. Attenuation of the liver parenchyma is diffusely decreased (D); axial and (E) coronal images show partial hypoattenuating thrombus at the origin of portal vein (*yellow arrow*).

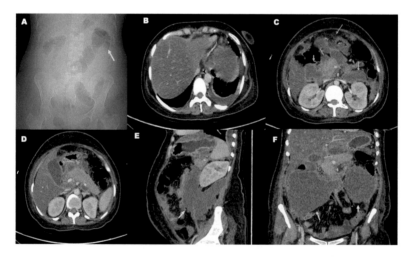

Figure 6.8 Acute pancreatitis with acute peripancreatic fluid collections: (A) abdominal X-ray AP view in supine position shows an abrupt transition from distended to collapsed colon just beyond the splenic flexure (colonic cut-off sign, *yellow arrow*). (B) Axial CECT shows left-sided mild pleural effusion (C) and (D) CECT axial images show diffusely enlarged homogenously enhancing pancreas with acute inflammatory fluid collections in the peripancreatic regions (*yellow arrow*), and gross mesenteric fat stranding (*green arrow*). The attenuation of liver parenchyma is diffusely decreased. (E) Sagittal and (F) coronal images show fluid collections in bilateral anterior, posterior renal fascia and extending below into combined fascia (*yellow arrow*).

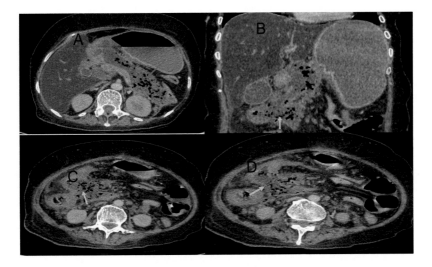

Figure 6.9 Acute necrotizing pancreatitis with colon perforation: 61-year-old patient with abdominal pain, distension, tenderness and unstable vitals. (A) Axial CECT shows near-total pancreas is replaced by inflammatory exudates in the region of head, body and tail (*blue arrow*), along with multiple internal gas densities within the collection. Peripancreatic collection is also seen extending into the lesser sac with edematous changes in the posterior wall of the stomach. Images (B, coronal), (C and D, axial) show a complete intramural defect in the transverse colon near hepatic flexure, which is seen communicating with the pancreatic necrotic collection suggesting perforation. There is severe surrounding mesenteric fat stranding.

- *CECT*: diagnostic modality of choice
  - Sensitivity: 100%; Specificity: 87%
  - Focal or diffuse parenchymal enlargement, indistinct pancreatic margin, peripancreatic fat stranding, with or without non-enhancing intraparenchymal/peripancreatic necrotic area, and collection (accumulates in lesser sac bilateral anterior pararenal space).

- *MRI*
  - Contrast-enhanced MR is equivalent to CT in the assessment of pancreatitis.

INTERSTITIAL EDEMATOUS PANCREATITIS

Focal or diffuse pancreatic enlargement, typically surrounded by peripancreatic inflammation or a small amount of fluid.
  - *On contrast-enhanced CT/MR imaging*: entire pancreas will enhance with no unenhanced area.
  - There may be surrounding fluid-containing collections but no peripancreatic necrotic collection should be there.

NECROTIZING PANCREATITIS

Three subtypes based on the location of the necrosis:
1. Pancreatic only
2. Peripancreatic only

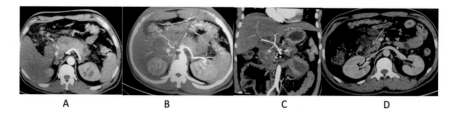

A	B	C	D

Figure 6.10 Pancreatitis-induced pseudoaneurysm formation: a 40-year-old male (known case of pancreatitis) presented with acute epigastric pain and generalized weakness. (A) Axial CECT image shows bulky pancreas with intrapancreatic necrotic collections (*dotted orange arrow*). A contrast-filled outpouching is noted in pancreatic head region (*solid blue arrow*). (B) Axial CECT MIP arterial phase shows the outpouching (*solid blue line*) arises from posterior superior pancreatico-duodenal artery. (C) Coronal CECT MIP arterial phase shows finding similar to image (B). (D) Axial CECT image shows a large rent in the second part of the duodenum (*solid green line*) with adjacent free intraperitoneal air foci, suggestive of duodenal perforation.

3. Combined pancreatic and peripancreatic: MC (non-enhancing pancreatic parenchyma along with non-enhancing peripancreatic necrotic collection, containing fluid with non-liquefied components)

Appendicitis

> What are the important abdominal imaging findings in appendicitis, cholecystitis, diverticulitis and abscess?

- Fecolith seen only in 35%, and no apparent cause is found in 65% of cases.
- In the early stages of inflamed fat, US is more sensitive than CT scan.
- Overall, CT is the most sensitive modality.

- **For Radiography:** insensitive

  - May show an *appendicolith* in 7–15% of cases.
  - *Mural thickening and displacement of caecal gas*: seen if an inflammatory phlegmon is present.

- **For USG**

  - *IOC in young patients*: Has sensitivity and specificity of 69% and 81%.
  - *Graded compression and sequential three-step patient positioning protocol*: initially examined in the conventional supine position > left posterior oblique position (45° LPO) > "second-look" supine position.
  - In the early stages of inflamed fat, US is more sensitive than CT scan.
  - *Diagnostic features*: aperistaltic, non-compressible, dilated appendix (>6 mm outer diameter), appears round when compression is applied with

surrounding echogenic prominent pericaecal and periappendiceal fat (usually >10 mm) and periappendiceal fluid collection or reactive nodal prominence. Hyperechoic appendicolith with posterior acoustic shadowing can be seen on sonography. If the wall layers are distinctly seen, then it implies that it's in the non-necrotic catarrhal or phlegmon stage. Loss of wall stratification with an irregular, asymmetrical echolucent contour indicates perforation or imminent perforation of the appendix (i.e. gangrenous stage). Wall thickening (3 mm or above) with mural hyperaemia is seen on Doppler examination. In the case of appendiceal abscess, the process of spontaneous evacuation of a pus collection to neighboring bowel can be followed by doing repeated US.

- **For CT**
  - Reported sensitivity 88–100%, specificity 91–99%.
  - *Diagnostic features*: divided into appendiceal, cecal and periappendiceal changes
  - Appendiceal changes are the same as seen on sonography. Focal wall non-enhancement represents gangrenous stage.
    - *Cecal changes*: include cecal apical thickening, the *arrowhead sign* (focal cecal wall thickening centered on the appendiceal orifice) and the *cecal bar sign* (inflammatory soft tissue at the base of the appendix that separates it from the contrast-filled cecum), both signs are visualized after rectal contrast administration.
    - *Periappendiceal inflammation* is noted in the form of fat stranding, thickening of the lateral conal fascia and mesoappendix, intraperitoneal fluid and mild lymph node enlargement. Appendiceal mass is seen on US and CT as a large mass of non-compressible fat around the appendix, often also with wall thickening of neighboring bowel loops. If there is a circumscribed pus collection, the diagnosis is appendiceal abscess. If not, the diagnosis is appendiceal phlegmon.

- **MRI:** done only as second modality after USG is equivocal in pregnant females.

ACUTE CHOLECYSTITIS

- **Plain radiography**: abdominal X-ray does not aid diagnosis of acute cholecystitis. Done as an initial evaluation to diagnose the complicated gall bladder disease. Only 15–20% of gallstones are visible on an X-ray. The key radiographic finding in emphysematous cholecystitis is air inside the gall bladder and/or in the gall bladder area (seen in 95% of patients) or in the biliary tree (15%); however, its absence on an abdominal radiograph does not exclude a diagnosis of emphysematous cholecystitis.
- **For sonography:** most accurate method to diagnose acute cholecystitis.
  - *Sensitivity and specificity* of ultrasound are approximately 88% and 80%, respectively.
  - *Diagnostic findings*: thickening of the gall bladder wall (>3 mm), distention of the gall bladder lumen (diameter >4/5 cm), gallstones with impacted

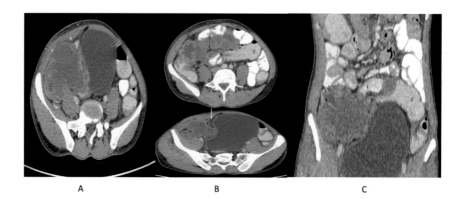

A   B   C

Figure 6.11 Perforated acute appendicitis with abscess: a 32-year-old male presented with acute abdomen, fever, nausea and vomiting. (A) Axial CECT image
showing a collection with thick, irregular, enhancing wall in right iliac fossa
surrounded by multiple bowel loops. Appendix was not separately visualized.
(B) Axial CECT at lower levels shows thickened wall of caecum and marked fat
stranding in omentum secondary to inflammatory changes, as well as there
is extension of the collection into anterior abdominal through a sinus tract.
(C) Coronal CECT showing large, thick-walled collection with irregular margin
abutting ileocaecal region.

stone in cystic duct or gall bladder neck, pericholecystic fluid collections
(multiple focal, non-contiguous, hypoechoic pockets of edema fluid within
the thickened wall are typically observed), positive sonographic Murphy
sign, hyperemic gall bladder wall on Doppler interrogation. (Hyperemia in
the gall bladder wall and the adjacent liver and a prominent cystic artery
are relatively specific findings in acute cholecystitis. Power Doppler has
been shown to be superior to color Doppler in detecting such hyperemia.)

Complications

Gall bladder stasis with bacterial overgrowth by 72 hours	Biliary sludge
Empyema of gall bladder	Heterogeneous luminal contents of variable echogenicity with layering
Increased pressure in gall bladder lumen and wall gangrene	Sloughed membranes; hypovascularity, loss of Murphy sign
Perforation	Loss of gourd shape; collection in or adjacent to gall bladder fossa

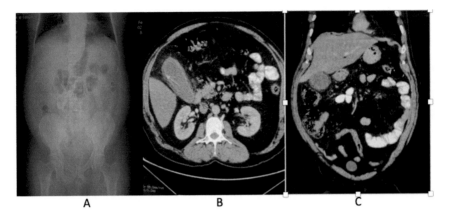

A   B   C

Figure 6.12 Acute acalculous cholecystitis in a 15-year-old male who presented with right upper quadrant pain. (A) X-ray abdomen in supine AP view appears normal. (B) Axial CECT abdomen image shows distended gall bladder with symmetrically thickened edematous wall and mural enhancement (*solid green line*). There is associated marked adjacent fat stranding surrounding the gall bladder fossa (*dotted blue line*) and few reactive lymph nodes (*solid blue line*). (C) Coronal CECT abdomen image in same patient reveals similar findings.

- ***Emphysematous cholecystitis***: its appearance on USG depends on the amount of gas present. Small amounts of gas appear as echogenic lines, with posterior dirty shadowing, reverberation, or ring-down artifact. A bright, echogenic line with posterior dirty shadowing is seen within the entire gall bladder fossa. Compression of the gall bladder fossa may help precipitate movement of gas bubbles. Pneumobilia may also be seen.

- ***Acalculous cholecystitis***: more common in critically ill patients, hence has worse prognosis. Its diagnosis can be difficult because gall bladder distention, wall thickening, internal sludge and pericholecystic fluid may all be present in critically ill patients without cholecystitis. Cholescintigraphy or percutaneous sampling of the luminal contents assist in the diagnosis. Ideally, there is non-visualization of the gall bladder.

- ***Chronic cholecystitis***: as a thick-walled gall bladder with gallstones. Differentiation from acute cholecystitis is made by the absence of other signs, namely, gall bladder distention, Murphy sign, and hyperemia in the wall.

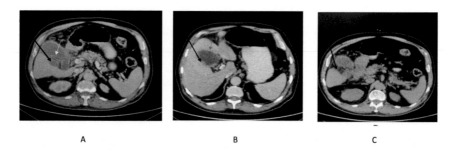

A   B   C

Figure 6.13 Acute gangrenous cholecystitis. A 46-year-old male presented with acute right upper quadrant pain abdomen with fever, nausea and vomiting. (A) Axial CECT image shows distended gall bladder with enhancing wall, mid-pericholecystic collection (*black solid arrow*) and a focal region of sloughed mucosa (*solid white arrow*). (B) Axial CECT image shows irregularly thickened enhancing (*black arrow*) and non-enhancing wall (*blue arrow*). (C) Axial CECT image shows extensive pericholecystic fat stranding (*black arrow*).

- **CT:** evidence of the diagnostic accuracy of CT is scarce and remains elusive.

  - *Diagnostic findings*: the presence of gallstones, gall bladder distension with diffuse wall thickening, increase in wall enhancement, and edema of pericholecystic fat.
    - Tensile gall bladder fundus sign (fundus bulging the anterior abdominal wall has ~75% sensitivity and ~95% specificity for acute cholecystitis in the absence of any other CT features). Transient pericholecystic liver rim enhancement may be seen.
    - CT signs suggesting *gangrenous cholecystitis* are gas in the wall or lumen, discontinuous and/or irregular mucosal enhancement internal membranes and pericholecystic abscess. Of these, interrupted wall enhancement is the most sensitive sign (70.6%) and is highly specific (100%).
    - CT findings of *emphysematous cholecystitis* show intramural and/or intraluminal gas caused.

- **MRI**

  - Sensitivity of 88% and specificity of 89%
  - Findings similar to those seen on ultrasound and CT. MR cholangiopancreatography (MRCP) may show an impacted stone in the gall bladder neck or cystic duct as a rounded filling defect.
  - The presence of one or more of the six criteria is indicative of acute cholecystitis:
    (1) gallstones, often impacted in the gall bladder neck or cystic duct
    (2) gall bladder wall thickening (>3 mm)
    (3) gall bladder wall edema
    (4) gall bladder distention (diameter > 40 mm)
    (5) pericholecystic fluid; and

(6) fluid around the liver, termed the "C sign" (small amount of fluid between the liver and the right hemidiaphragm or the abdominal wall, different from pericholecystic fluid)

ACUTE DIVERTICULTIS

Inflammation of colonic diverticula, in a **true diverticulum** (more frequently noted in *right*-sided diverticulitis) or in a **false or pseudo-diverticulum** (generally noted in *left*-sided diverticulitis)

- **Plain radiography**
  - Is of little value in the assessment of suspected diverticulitis. May be used to demonstrate free intraperitoneal air from perforation, portal venous gas or signs of bowel ileus or obstruction. However, these findings are nonspecific.
  - The small, contained perforations cannot be demonstrated on these, which are commonly encountered on computed tomography (CT).
  - Is not sensitive for other complications such as abscess and fistula.
- **USG**
  - Sensitivity: 77–98%; Specificity: 80–99%
  - *Diagnostic features*: at least one diverticulum; seen as bright bowel outpouching (bowel bright "ears") showing some degree of acoustic shadowing due to the presence of gas or inspissated feces. Echogenic and non-compressible fat surrounding the diverticula suggesting an inflammatory process of the surrounding fat planes. Bowel wall thickening (>4 mm). **Target sign or pseudokidney sign** (the hypoechoic wall surrounding a hyperechoic center) may be seen. If abscess is seen in the form of organized collection, it mandates further CT evaluation.
- **Contrast enema**
  - Sensitivity: 80–92%
  - Barium enema should not performed in the acute setting due to the risk of perforation and peritonitis.
  - Also causes artifacts that may preclude diagnosis of a CT scan.
  - *Diagnostic findings*: fold thickening, segmental spasm, sinus tract, fistula, mass effect from abscess and extraluminal free or contained contrast may be demonstrated and can be diagnostic of acute diverticulitis.
  - Is more useful for chronic diverticulitis.
- **CT**
  - High sensitivity of 94%; Specificity of 99%
  - *CT abdomen and pelvis with oral, intravenous (IV) contrast and/or colonic contrast*: diagnostic modality of choice in the setting of left lower quadrant pain with or without fever, except in women of childbearing age, when ultrasound (US) is the initial preferred modality for unexplained left lower quadrant pain.
    - *Oral contrast* is used mostly; however, contrast does not reach up to sigmoid colon by the time examination is done.
    - *IV contrast* helps identify abscess and enhancement of colonic wall. Hence is used unless contraindicated.

- *Oral contrast* may not be necessary, helps to distend colon, detect fistulous tracts and increase the accuracy of examination.
- *Diagnostic findings*: colonic wall thickening (wall thickness > 3 mm on the short axis of the lumen), disproportionate pericolic fat stranding are the most frequent signs. Inflamed diverticulum along with enhancement of colonic wall can be seen.
- Complicated diverticulitis are easily demonstrated on CECT.
  - Diverticular perforation
    - Extravasation of gas and fluid into pelvis and peritoneal cavity
  - Abscess formation (seen in up to 30% of cases)
    - Seen as a fluid-containing mass with or without air and an enhancing wall
  - Fistula formation (usually a chronic complication)
    - Gas in the bladder
    - Direct visualization of a fistulous tract
  - Others: bowel obstruction, hepatic abscess and inferior mesenteric vein thrombosis
- Patients with abscesses <3 cm: manage conservatively, and those with abscesses >3 cm: benefit from percutaneous drainage with referral for surgical follow-up.
- Prior to catheter removal, a tube injection with iodinated contrast performed under fluoroscopy is recommended to exclude communication with the colon. Even in cases where communication to the colon is documented, continued percutaneous drainage can result in resolution of the fistula without surgical intervention.
- **MRI**
  - Sensitivity: 86–94%; Specificity: 88–92%
  - Findings are similar to that of CT.

PNEUMOPERITONEUM

- **Plain radiograph**: An erect chest X-ray is the most sensitive for the detection of free intraperitoneal gas.
  - Sensitivity of 79%, specificity of 64%
  - *Diagnostic signs*:
    - *Subdiaphragmatic free gas* (even 1 mL of free gas can be detected, but the patient may have to be kept in upright position for about 10 minutes for the gas to rise).
    - *Continuous diaphragm sign* (seen in large amount of free subphrenic gas).
      - *Leaping dolphin sign*, aka the diaphragm muscle slip sign (on supine abdominal radiograph), requires large amount of free intraperitoneal gas, and represents the outlining of the diaphragmatic muscle slips by free intraperitoneal gas.
        - The *cupola sign* (on a supine chest/abdominal radiograph) refers to gas underneath the central tendon of the diaphragm in the midline.

- *Diagnostic signs on abdominal radiograph in supine position*:
  - *Rigler sign*: gas is outlining both sides of the bowel wall, i.e. from within the bowel lumen and outside the bowel wall due to pneumoperitoneum, it is seen when > 1000 mL of pneumoperitoneum is present.
  - The *telltale triangle sign* or *triangle sign* or *telltale triangle* (seen in supine, cross-table lateral or decubitus view) represents the appearance of a radiolucent triangle of gas formed between three loops of bowel or between two loops of bowel and the abdominal wall.
  - Football sign: seen in massive pneumoperitoneum; abdominal cavity is outlined by gas with median umbilical ligament and falciform ligament representing the sutures of the football.
  - The *falciform ligament sign/silver sign* (seen in large pneumoperitoneum), falciform ligament is outlined with free abdominal gas.
  - The *inverted "V" sign/lateral umbilical ligament sign (in supine position)*, visualization of an inverted "V" shape in the pelvis, represents free gas outlining the lateral umbilical ligaments.
  - The *urachus sign*, free abdominal gas outlines the median umbilical ligament.
  - The *fissure for ligamentum teres sign or extrahepatic ligamentum teres sign*: free abdominal gas outline the ligaments teres.
  - The *lucent liver sign* represent reduction of hepatic radiodensity due to collection of free intraperitoneal gas located anterior to the liver.

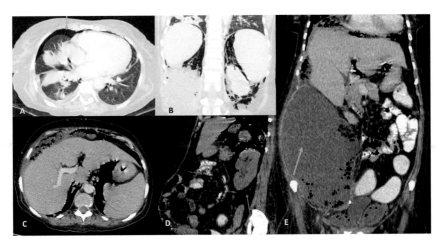

Figure 6.14 Pneumothorax and pneumoretroperitoneum. (A) Axial HRCT thorax lung window shows air in the right pleural space (*blue arrow*). Coronal (B), axial (C) and sagittal (D) abdominal computed tomography images show gas collections dissecting along the retroperitoneum in the perirenal space along the kidney, aorta and psoas muscle suggesting perforation in retroperitoneum (*orange arrows*). (E) A large collection with air-fluid level in the right paracolic gutter indicating a gas-containing abscess is suggestive of retroperitoneal abscess (*green arrow*).

- The *doge cap sign/Morrison pouch sign* is a triangular-shaped (although may also be crescentic or semicircular) gas lucency, bounded by the 11th rib in the right upper quadrant due to air in the Morrison pouch.
- The *periportal free gas sign* is strongly suggestive for upper gastrointestinal tract perforation.

- **Ultrasonography**
  - A linear-array transducer (10–12 MHz) is more sensitive than a standard curvilinear abdominal transducer (2–5 MHz).
  - Sensitivity of 93%; Specificity of 64%
  - Ultrasound is more sensitive than plain radiograph to diagnose pneumoperitoneum.
  - *Diagnostic signs*: peritoneal stripe sign is enhancement of the peritoneal stripe either with or without long-path reverberation artifacts, which extend into the far field. Discrete, hyperechoic foci representing gas bubbles are often associated with short-path reverberation artifacts, which appear as comet tails, or if tapering, ring down artifacts. Gas may also cluster in a manner that results in an underlying non-homogenous (or dirty) acoustic shadow. Free intraperitoneal air moves with the patient position. Gas gets displaced with caudal pressure on the probe above the collection and reappears with cessation of the pressure.

FURTHER READING

1. Rudralingam V, Footitt C, Layton B. Ascites matters. *Ultrasound.* 2017;25:69–79.
2. Laméris W, van Randen A, van Es HW, van Heesewijk JP, van Ramshorst B, Bouma WH, et al. Imaging strategies for detection of urgent conditions in patients with acute abdominal pain: Diagnostic accuracy study. *BMJ.* 2009;338:b2431.
3. Barker CS, Lindsell DR. Ultrasound of the palpable abdominal mass. *Clin Radiol.* 1990;41:98–9.
4. Stapakis JC, Thickman D. Diagnosis of pneumoperitoneum: Abdominal CT vs. upright chest film. *J Comput Assist Tomogr.* 1992;16:713–16.
5. Mallo RD, Salem L, Lalani T, Flum DR. Computed tomography diagnosis of ischemia and complete obstruction in small bowel obstruction: A systematic review. *J Gastrointest Surg.* 2005;9:690–4.
6. Chernyak V, Fowler KJ. Introduction to the special section on quantitative imaging. *Abdom Radiol.* 2022, https://doi.org/10.1007/s00261-022-03637-8.

7

The pregnant patient

SMITA MANCHANDA, SURABHI VYAS
AND ASHISH VERMA

INTRODUCTION

- The common indications for admission in the ICU setting are pregnancy-associated life-threatening complications such as antepartum and post-partum haemorrhage (APH & PPH), hypertensive disorders of pregnancy (eclampsia, pre-eclampsia and pregnancy-induced hypertension), trauma and sepsis.
- Some less severe complications such as torsion of ovarian cysts and red degeneration of leiomyomas may also require admission.
- Septic abortions, ectopic pregnancy and multiple pregnancies may occasionally require ICU admission.

COMMON DISEASE ENTITIES

Post-partum haemorrhage

- Post-partum haemorrhage (PPH) can occur following a normal delivery or caesarean section and is a leading cause of maternal morbidity.
- Primary (early) PPH occurs within 24 hours after delivery and are mostly caused due to uterine atony, lower genital tract lacerations, uterine dehiscence, retained products of conception (RPOC) and coagulation abnormalities.
- Secondary (late) PPH occurs 24 hours to 12 weeks after delivery and is most commonly caused by RPOC, infection, placental site subinvolution and coagulopathy.
- *Clinical:* severe bleeding may also be complicated by disseminated intravascular coagulopathy (DIC), abdominal compartment syndrome, renal failure and adult respiratory distress syndrome.

DOI: 10.1201/9781003218739-7

UTERINE ATONY

Uterine atony is the lack of uterine contraction after delivery and is one of the most common causes of PPH. Large uterus size with heavy vaginal bleeding is the typical presentation.

Imaging

- *USG*: large uterus with internal echogenic blood clots.
- *CT*: enlarged post-partum uterus with hematoma within. Intravenous or intra-arterial contrast material extravasation can be seen on CECT.

PUERPERAL GENITAL HEMATOMA

Puerperal genital hematomas are relatively rare and can result from birth canal trauma or episiotomy trauma. These can be classified as vulvovaginal, vulvar, paravaginal and supravaginal hematomas.

Imaging

- *USG*: hematomas are seen as heterogenous lesions with no internal vascularity on color Doppler imaging.
- *CT*: the exact extent of a hematoma is well depicted on CT with accurate demonstration of paravesical, presacral or pararectal extensions.

RETAINED PRODUCTS OF CONCEPTION (RPOC)

These are more commonly seen after termination of pregnancy than after normal vaginal or post-caesarean deliveries. RPOC is the most common cause of secondary PPH presenting as pelvic pain and bleeding. It refers to intrauterine tissue of trophoblastic origin developing after conception/pregnancy and persisting after delivery or termination.

Imaging

In situations where imaging suggests RPOC (Figure 7.1), a careful evaluation of the clinical details, serum β-hCG levels is essential in the differentiation of RPOC from uterine AVM and gestational trophoblastic neoplasia.

- *USG*: reveals an echogenic mass within the endometrial cavity with various degrees of vascularity on color Doppler US. The flow is high velocity and low-resistance flow.
- *MRI*: reveals an endometrial polypoidal mass with heterogeneous signal intensity on T1- and T2-weighted images. Contrast enhancement can be variable depending on the vascularity of the RPOCs.

UTERINE ARTERY PSEUDOANEURYSM

The incidence of uterine artery pseudoaneurysm is low (approximately 3% of severe PPHs), and it is a potentially life-threatening condition. Pseudoaneurysms usually result from laceration or injury of the arterial wall associated with surgical procedures such as caesarean delivery, and dilatation and curettage result

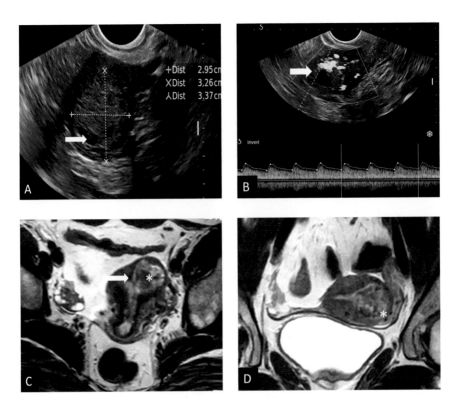

Figure 7.1 Highly vascular retained products of conception (RPOC). A 32-year-old female presented with excessive bleeding post-dilatation and curettage (D&C) 1 month prior (Beta-hCG level 50 mLU/mL). (A) TVS shows a heterogeneously hyperechoic focal lesion with anechoic spaces in the endometrial cavity and myometrium of uterine fundus (*arrow*). (B) Color Doppler image shows high vascularity within the lesion, with low-resistance arterial flow in the anechoic spaces (*arrow*). (C) Axial T2-weighted MRI image shows focal distension of left supero-lateral endometrial cavity (*arrow*), with heterogenous content and flow voids within (*), associated with the obliteration of junctional zone and thinning of the myometrium. (D) Coronal T2-weighted MRI image shows multiple flow voids within the lesion (*).

in uterine artery pseudoaneurysms. During vaginal delivery, injury may be to the vaginal artery or obturator artery, whereas in caesarean delivery it usually involves the uterine artery.

Imaging

- *USG*: pseudoaneurysm is typically seen as an anechoic or hypoechoic intra-uterine lesion with intense vascularity on color Doppler US (Figure 7.2). Spectral Doppler USG reveals turbulent, bidirectional systolic and diastolic flow with aliasing.

- *CT*: CT angiography shows the arterial pseudoaneurysm with anatomical delineation (Figure 7.2).
- *MRI*: pseudoaneurysm is seen as a flow void on T2-weighted images with intense post-contrast enhancement on gadolinium-enhanced T1-weighted images. Pre-gadolinium T1-weighted images may reveal a hyperintense

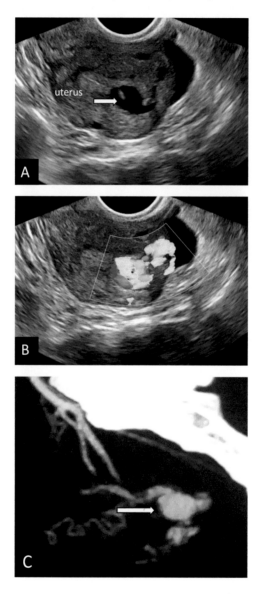

Figure 7.2 Uterine artery pseudoaneurysm. A 20-year-old female with excessive bleeding post-dilatation and curettage for incomplete abortion. (A) TVS shows anechoic lacuna in subendometrial location (*arrow*). (B) On color Doppler evaluation, there was intense to-and-fro flow. (C) CT angiography revealed hypertrophied left uterine artery and rounded pseudoaneurysm (*arrow*).

hematoma surrounding the lesion. Dilatation and curettage is contraindicated in these cases, and transcatheter arterial embolization is the treatment of choice for uterine artery pseudoaneurysm.

UTERINE ARTERIOVENOUS MALFORMATIONS (AVMs)

These can be congenital or acquired. Congenital AVMs present as women of childbearing age with spontaneous abortions. Acquired AVMs present as excessive bleeding (continuous or intermittent) in women with a predisposing cause such as post-dilatation and curettage, uterine surgery, or infection. The β-hCG levels are negative in these cases.

Imaging

- *USG*: USG reveals multiple tubular, anechoic or hypoechoic areas within the myometrium, which show intensely vascular, multidirectional high-velocity flow and a mosaic pattern of color signal. There is evidence of low-resistance flow with low pulsatility of the arterial waveform, and pulsatile high-velocity venous waveform (Figure 7.3).
- *CT/MRI*: Cross-sectional imaging reveals a vascular lesion with myometrial involvement. Early venous return is noted at CECT and multiple flow voids within the mass on MRI.
- *DSA*: There is evidence of a tortuous, hypertrophic arterial mass with large accessory feeding vessels, bilateral hypertrophy of uterine arteries and early drainage into enlarged hypertrophic veins. Uterine artery embolization is used for treating the AVMs and also when the vascular malformations are a part of RPOC. UAE is considered if the PSV of the lesion is high (≥ 60–70 cm/s).

Puerperal sepsis

Puerperal sepsis is a leading cause of maternal mortality responsible for approximately 15% of all maternal deaths.

Puerperal sepsis was defined by the WHO (in 1992) as an infection of the genital tract which can occur at any time between the rupture of membranes (ROM) or labour and the 42nd day post-partum with two or more of the following symptoms: pelvic pain, abnormal vaginal discharge, fever and delay in the reduction of the size of the uterus.

- *Clinical*: the signs and symptoms of sepsis can be obscured by the physiological changes of pregnancy and puerperium. A high level of clinical suspicion is needed for an early diagnosis and prompt treatment. The common clinical manifestations include fever with chills or rigours, diarrhea or vomiting, rash, abdominal/pelvic pain and tenderness, offensive vaginal discharge, productive cough, urinary symptoms, breast engorgement/redness, wound infection, delay in uterine involution, heavy lochia, non-specific signs such as lethargy and reduced appetite.
- *Imaging*: puerperal sepsis is a clinical diagnosis with imaging having only a supportive role to play. Imaging is targeted at the suspected site of clinical

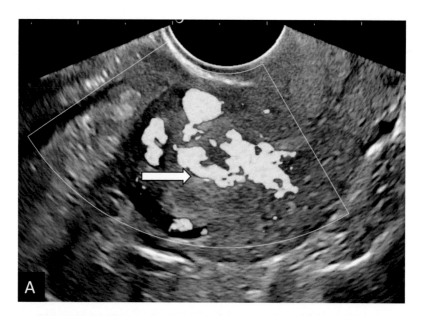

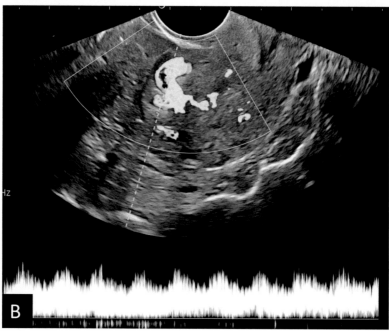

Figure 7.3 Uterine arteriovenous malformation. A 30-year-old female with excessive bleeding post-dilatation and curettage for spontaneous abortion. (A) Color Doppler image shows a mosaic pattern of color signal (*arrow*) within an ill-defined lesion in the endometrial cavity and anterior myometrium. (B) Spectral analysis of the color flow shows pulsatile high-velocity venous waveform.

evaluation. For example, ultrasound breast for evaluation of suspected mastitis/ breast abscess, ultrasound abdomen for scar-related complications, collections, cystitis and pyelonephritis. Further cross-sectional imaging may be done in the form of CT or MRI as required.

- *USG breast*: inflammatory changes in the form of an ill-defined hypoechoic area with peripheral hyperechogenecity may represent mastitis. Breast abscess is seen as a multilocular hypoechoic collection with peripheral vascularity (Figure 7.4). There is no internal vascularity, and the lesion displays through transmission.
- *In cases of cystitis,* USG of the bladder reveals internal mobile debris within the bladder lumen, and the bladder wall thickness may be increased (Figure 7.5). Focal, hypoechoic areas with reduced areas of cortical vascularity and internal echoes within the pelvicalyceal system are suggestive of acute pyelonephritis.
- *Scar-related complications*: scar rupture (usually with a previous history of lower caesarean segment scar) is characterized by separation of all layers of the uterine wall, including the membrane, decidua, myometrium and serosa. There is thus direct communication between the uterine cavity and the peritoneal cavity.
  - CECT reveals focal disruption of the uterine wall, broad ligament hematoma and hemoperitoneum. Hypoattenuating fluid with or without air bubbles may be seen in the endometrial cavity and the scar site with extrauterine extension. Scar dehiscence may be seen as a focal disruption of the uterine myometrium. There is an ill-defined hypoattenuating lesion within the densely enhancing myometrium, but the serosal margin is intact (Figure 7.6).
  - MRI, with its inherent superior contrast resolution, is the ideal imaging modality to differentiate between scar dehiscence and scar rupture.

Adnexal torsion during pregnancy

Adnexal torsion during pregnancy is a gynecological emergency. It is very rare, with a reported incidence of 0.2–3%. It refers to a partial or complete rotation of the adnexa around the ligamentous supports.

- *Clinical:* usually seen in the first and early second trimesters and presents as acute abdomen. Torsion may be of the ovary or any pre-existing lesion such as a dermoid cyst.
- *Imaging:*
  - USG: enlarged, hypoechoic ovary with follicles situated in the periphery is characteristic. Twisting of the vascular pedicle along with thickened pedicle is commonly identified.
    - *Color Doppler* evaluation can depict the internal color flow within the torted ovary.

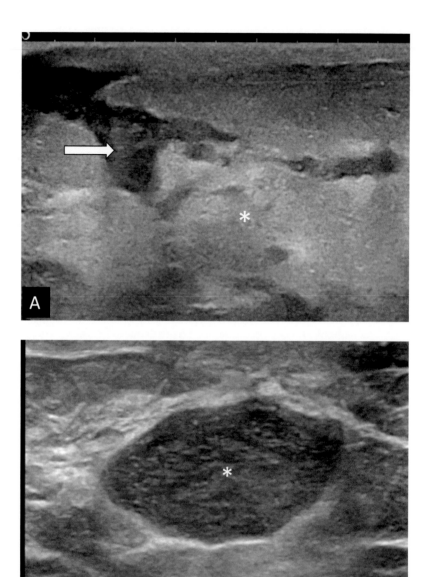

Figure 7.4 Mastitis/breast abscess. (A) USG breast reveals ill-defined areas of altered echotexture with hyperechogenicity (*) and tracking abscess (*arrow*). (B) USG in another patient shows a lobulated cystic lesion with mobile internal echoes (*). Aspiration revealed purulent material suggestive of infected galactocele.

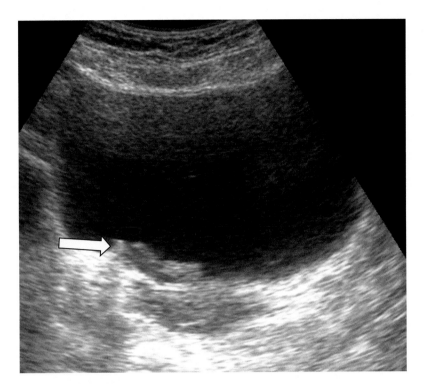

Figure 7.5 Cystitis. Axial USG image reveals mobile internal debris in the urinary bladder (*arrow*).

Red degeneration of leiomyoma

Degeneration of leiomyomas (hyaline, cystic, red or calcific) is common. However, during pregnancy, red or carneous degeneration is the most common form of degeneration. It is a type of hemorrhagic infarction of the leiomyoma and occurs secondary to venous thrombosis in periphery of the tumour.

- *Clinical:* the patient may present in emergency with varying degrees of abdominal pain, along with systemic symptoms such as fever and leukocytosis.
- *Imaging*
  - *USG:* enlargement of the leiomyoma with heterogenous appearance is seen.
  - *MRI:* the peripheral high-T1 signal-intensity rim is very characteristic, and T2 signal intensity is variable with or without a low-signal-intensity rim.

First trimester complications

- **Ectopic Pregnancy**
  Implantation of a fertilized ovum outside the endometrial cavity of the uterus is known as ectopic pregnancy. Ectopic pregnancies are seen in about 1.4% of all pregnancies and are responsible for 15% of pregnancy-related deaths. Rupture of an ectopic pregnancy is potentially life-threatening. It results in irregular, crenated margins of the lesion, pelvic hematoma and hemoperitoneum.

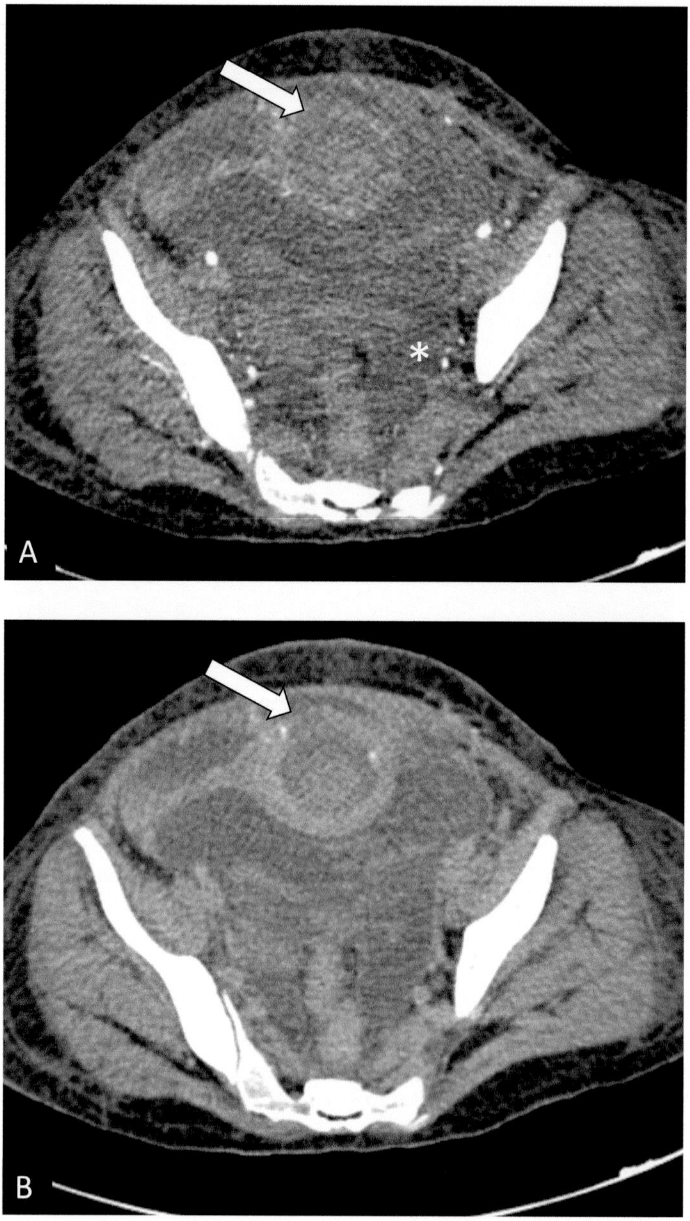

Figure 7.6 Scar dehiscence. Axial (A) CECT reveal focal thinning and discontinuity in the anterior myometrium (*arrow*) at the lower uterine segment with ascites (*). (B) Delayed CECT image shows the serosa to be intact (*arrow*).

- *Clinical:* a triad of abdominal or pelvic pain, vaginal bleeding, along with an adnexal mass is the classical presentation. Symptoms can also be non-specific including amenorrhea, adnexal tenderness, cervical motion tenderness and vague pain abdomen. A raised β-hCG level is seen in ectopic pregnancies, but normal levels do not rule out a chronic ectopic pregnancy. The ectopic pregnancy can be tubal, interstitial, cervical or ovarian in location.
- *Imaging:* transvaginal USG is the investigation of choice. A complex adnexal mass is seen separate from the ovary. The adnexal lesion can be a cyst with internal yolk sac and embryo and a thick hyperechoic ring surrounding the extrauterine gestational sac (Figure 7.7). Peripheral hypervascularity of the hyperechoic ring is known as the "ring of fire sign" and represents high-velocity, low-impedance flow surrounding the pregnancy. Probe tenderness can also be elicited during the transvaginal examination.

- **Ovarian hyperstimulation syndrome (OHSS)**
  OHSS is a rare but occasionally life-threatening complication of infertility treatment. OHSS is characterized by cystic enlargement of bilateral ovaries and a fluid shift from the intravascular compartment to the third space due to ovarian neoangiogenesis and increased capillary permeability. Spontaneous OHSS occurs because of non-iatrogenic ovarian stimulation in spontaneous cycles and is seen in cases of gestational trophoblastic tumour, pituitary adenomas, hypothyroidism and β-hCG-secreting tumours.
  - *Clinical:* abdominal pain, decreased urine output, bloating, nausea, vomiting, diarrhea, dyspnea and pedaledema are typically seen. OHSS is classified according to the Modified Golan classification into three categories and five grades.
    - Mild OHSS includes abdominal distention and discomfort (grade 1) and nausea, vomiting and/or diarrhea with ovarian enlargement from 5 to 12 cm along with grade 1 disease (grade 2).
      - Moderate OHSS includes mild OHSS plus USG evidence of ascites (grade 3).
      - Severe OHSS is characterized by the features of moderate OHSS plus clinical evidence of ascites and/or hydrothorax and breathing difficulties (grade 4). Grade 5 disease includes the changes of grade 4 diseases along with a change in the blood volume, increased blood viscosity due to haemoconcentration, coagulation abnormalities and diminished renal perfusion and function.
  - *Imaging*
    - USG (Figure 7.8): there is bilateral symmetric enlargement of ovaries (often >12 cm in size), with multiple cysts of varying sizes (classic spoke-wheel appearance). The presence of ascites and pleural along with pericardial effusion are worse prognostic indicators.
    - *CT/MRI*: Enlarged ovaries with bilateral cysts and ascites along with pleural and pericardial effusion are noted.

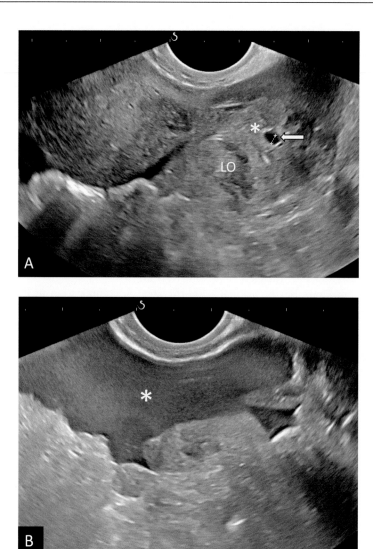

Figure 7.7. Ectopic pregnancy. (A) TVS image reveals a complex echogenic mass (*) in the left adnexa adjacent to the left ovary (LO). An internal gestational sac-like structure (*arrow*) is present. (B) Moderate hemoperitoneum was also seen (*).

CONCLUSION

Ultrasonography is the imaging modality of choice, especially for bedside evaluation in an emergency setting. The imaging findings need to be interpreted with the laboratory findings in an appropriate clinical scenario.

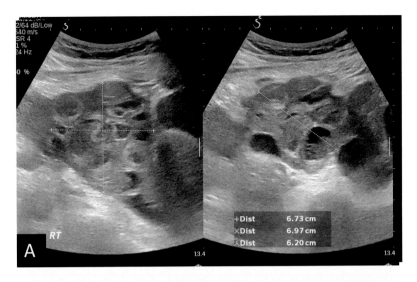

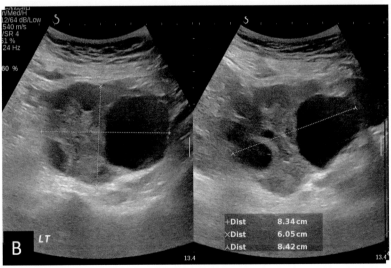

Figure 7.8 Ovarian Hyperstimulation Syndrome (OHSS). A 31-year-old female on ovulation induction therapy presented with acute pain abdomen, nausea and vomiting. (A, B) TVS dual mode shows enlarged bilateral ovaries with multiple cysts of varying sizes.

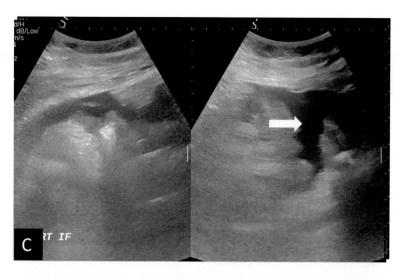

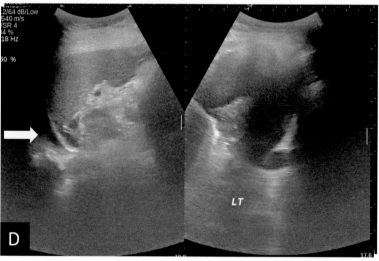

Figure 7.8 (Continued) (C) Free fluid (*arrow*) is noted in the right iliac fossa. (D) Mild left pleural effusion (*arrow*) is also noted.

FURTHER READING

1. Pollock W, Rose L, Dennis CL. Pregnant and postpartum admissions to the intensive care unit: A systematic review. *Intensive Care Med.* 2010 Sep;36(9):1465–74, doi: 10.1007/s00134-010-1951-0. Epub 2010 July 15. PMID: 20631987.
2. Lee NK, Kim S, Lee JW, Sol YL, Kim CW, Hyun Sung K, Jang HJ, Suh DS. Postpartum hemorrhage: Clinical and radiologic aspects. *Eur J Radiol.* 2010 Apr;74(1):50–9, doi: 10.1016/j.ejrad.2009.04.062. Epub 2009 May 23. PMID: 19477095.
3. Iraha Y, Okada M, Toguchi M, Azama K, Mekaru K, Kinjo T, Kudaka W, Aoki Y, Aoyama H, Matsuzaki A, Murayama S. Multimodality imaging in secondary

postpartum or postabortion hemorrhage: Retained products of conception and related conditions. *Jpn J Radiol.* 2018 Jan;36(1):12–22, doi: 10.1007/s11604-017-0687-y. Epub 2017 Oct 19. PMID: 29052024.

4. Laifer-Narin SL, Kwak E, Kim H, Hecht EM, Newhouse JH. Multimodality imaging of the postpartum or posttermination uterus: Evaluation using ultrasound, computed tomography, and magnetic resonance imaging. *Curr Probl Diagn Radiol.* 2014;43(6):374–85.

5. Sadan O, Golan A, Girtler O, et al. Role of sonography in the diagnosis of retained products of conception. *J Ultrasound Med.* 2004;23:371–4.

6. McGonegle SJ, Dziedzic TS, Thomas J, Hertzberg BS. Pseudoaneurysm of the uterine artery after an uncomplicated spontaneous vaginal delivery. *J Ultrasound Med.* 2006;25(12):1593–7.

7. Timmerman D, Wauters J, Van Calenbergh S, Van Schou- broeck D, Maleux G, Van Den Bosch T, et al. Color Doppler imaging is a valuable tool for the diagnosis and management of uterine vascular malformations. *Ultrasound Obstet Gynecol.* 2003;21(6):570–7.

8. Timor-Tritsch IE, Haynes MC, Monteagudo A, Khatib N, Kovács S. Ultrasound diagnosis and management of acquired uterine enhanced myometrial vascularity/arteriovenous malformations. *Am J Obstet Gynecol.* 2016;214(6):731.e1–731.e10, doi: 10.1016/j.ajog.2015.12.024.

9. Buddeberg BS, Aveling W. Puerperal sepsis in the 21st century: Progress, new challenges and the situation worldwide. *Postgrad Med J.* 2015;91:572–8.

10. Has R, Topuz S, Kalelioglu I, Tagrikulu D. Imaging features of postpartum uterine rupture: A case report. *Abdom Imaging.* 2008;33:101–3.

11. Wang Y, Deng, S. Clinical characteristics, treatment and outcomes of adnexal torsion in pregnant women: A retrospective study. *BMC Pregnancy Childbirth.* 2020;20:483, doi.org/10.1186/s12884-020-03173-7.

12. Kawakami S, Togashi K, Konishi I, Kimura I, Fukuoka M, Mori T, Konishi J. Red degeneration of uterine leiomyoma: MR appearance. *J Comput Assist Tomogr.* 1994 Nov–Dec;18(6):925–8, doi: 10.1097/00004728-199411000-00014. PMID: 7962801.

13. Petrides A, Dinglas C, Chavez M, Taylor S, Mahboob S. Revisiting ectopic pregnancy: A pictorial essay. *J Clin Imaging Sci.* 2014 July 31;4:37, doi: 10.4103/2156-7514.137817. PMID: 25161806; PMCID: PMC4142466.

14. Histed SN, Deshmukh M, Masamed R, Jude CM, Mohammad S, Patel MK. Ectopic pregnancy: A trainee's guide to making the right call: Women's imaging. *Radiographics.* 2016 Nov–Dec;36(7):2236–7, doi: 10.1148/rg.2016160080. PMID: 27831839.

15. Golan A, Ron-el R, Herman A, Soffer Y, Weinraub Z, Caspi E. Ovarian hyperstimulation syndrome: An update review. *Obstet Gynecol Surv.* 1989;44:430–40.

8

Pediatric imaging

ISHAN KUMAR, ASHISH VERMA AND
ANIRBAN HOM CHOUDHURI

IMAGING MODALITIES AND TECHNICAL CONSIDERATIONS

- Emphasis is placed on using the modalities with low or no radiation.
- X-ray and fluoroscopy, including barium studies, intravenous urography, urethrography (retrograde or micturating urethrography), digital subtraction angiography and CT scans, use ionizing radiation. MRI and ultrasound utilize no ionizing radiation.
- Adverse effects of radiation include dose-independent (stochastic) effects such as carcinogenesis, genetic effects as well as dose-dependent effects such as cataracts, skin/hair changes, diarrhea and sterility.
- Image Gently Campaign: a global campaign for optimizing the radiation parameters and using dedicated pediatric imaging protocols (CT and fluoroscopy).
- ALARA (As Low As Reasonably Achievable) concept is central to the practice of pediatric radiology.
- Principles of dose reduction
  - *Justification*: it is the clinician's responsibility to ensure that the examination (utilizing radiation) is actually indicated and justified. ACR Appropriateness Criteria and Practice Guidelines should be followed.
  - *Optimization*: the clinician and radiologist should be aware about the child's radiation history, should adjust CT parameters according to child size, region/organ scanned and indication (e.g. low-dose head CT protocol). Multiphasic scans (e.g. NCCT, arterial/portal/venous phase) should be avoided unless absolutely necessary. Radiation dose of each scan should be recorded (CT dose should be recorded as dose length product [DLP]).

DOI: 10.1201/9781003218739-8

- *Dose limitation*: the total dose to any individual should not exceed the appropriate limits.

X-ray

- *Chest X-ray* is the most commonly used imaging exam in pediatric imaging of pneumonia, airway disease, birth abnormalities, trauma and swallowed foreign bodies.
- *Abdominal X-ray* is often the first exam used to evaluate the source of acute pain in the abdominal region such as kidney stones, intestinal obstruction or perforation and swallowed foreign objects.
- *Bone X-rays* are used to diagnose fractures, infection and bone tumors.
- *Fluoroscopy* uses continuous X-rays to see internal organs in motion, especially used in gastrointestinal dye (barium studies) to diagnose tracheoesophageal fistula, bowel obstruction in infants due to congenital causes, Hirschsprung disease, malrotation etc.
- *Intravenous urography*: serial X-ray of kidneys after giving iodinated IV contrast to demonstrate stones, strictures in pelvicalyceal system, ureters and urinary bladder.
- *Retrograde (RGU) and micturating urethrography (MCU)*: direct administration of iodinated contrast into the urethra and urinary bladder to demonstrate anterior and posterior urethral stricture/injury or vescicoureteric reflux.
- *Technical aspects* should be discussed with the radiologist/radiography technicians to optimize and use the lowest radiation dose possible while producing the best images for evaluation.
  - Reduce field size: avoid long bones while taking abdominal/chest radiograph as it contains red marrow.
  - Optimize collimation, especially in infants and young children. Collimation reduces the volume of tissue irradiated and decreases patient exposure but requires a radiographer's dedication and awareness.
  - Use highest possible KV, at least 60 KV for head, body and trunk.
  - Shielding of gonads is necessary.

Computed tomography

- *Chest CT* (Table 8.1): use low-dose 25–75 mA for lung window, 50–75 mA for mediastinal (67% dose reduction compared to conventional 240 MA). HRCT: use low-dose technique, <100 mA (preferably 40 mA). Interslice spacing can be varied depending on the pathology suspected. Discuss the need for reduction of dose with CT technician. Record the radiation dose received (Unit: dose length product).
- *Brain CT*: use 125–150 mA instead of 250 mA. In neonates, 30% of marrow is in skull, hence marrow-absorbed dose in a child < 6 years is higher than chest/abdomen CT.

Table 8.1 Suggested Tube Current for Chest and Abdominal CT for Children of Different Age Groups

Weight (kg)	Chest (mA)	Abdomen (mA)
5–9	40	60
9–18	50	70
18–27	60	80
27–36	70	100
36–45	80	120

Ultrasound

- Point-of-care ultrasound (POCUS), i.e. bedside ultrasound, has become an essential tool for clinical practice in recent years, especially in the ICU setting.
  - It can be performed quickly and at the bedside (so that patients need not be moved), and it also allows serial imaging.
  - Although mainly practiced by radiologists, it has been decades since ultrasonography became an indispensable technique in intensive care training.
  - Table 8.2 summarizes the indications and findings of POCUS in pediatric care.

CHEST AND AIRWAYS

Imaging modalities

X-ray neck: in patients with inspiratory stridor/suspected upper respiratory disease, soft tissue neck X-ray. Standard soft tissue neck radiographic views consist of both an anteroposterior (AP) view and a lateral view with extended neck. An additional expiratory lateral view of the neck subsequently may be obtained for assessment of subglottic stenosis.

Chest radiography: AP view should be done in infants and young children (<5 years). In older children, PA views to be done (lateral view if required).

ULTRASOUND

- To characterize a peripheral lung opacity (parenchymal versus pleural disease)
- To characterize pleural fluid (simple or complex)
- To diagnose pneumothorax
- To provide ultrasound-guided drainage, biopsy

COMPUTED TOMOGRAPHY

- *Non-CCT study* is performed mainly to assess a fixed airway narrowing or stenosis.

Table 8.2 Indications and Findings of POCUS in Pediatric Care

Clinical Indication	Diagnosis	Findings
Hemodynamic assessment	Hypovolemic shock	Small IVC diameter that collapses with inspiration, small cardiac chambers
	Compromised LV systolic function	Enlarged left ventricle, decreased overall systolic motion of LV, dilated IVC with reduced respiratory changes
	Pericardium	Effusion
		Compression of heart chambers
Respiratory assessment	Pleural effusion	Anechoic (dark) fluid, quantification and guided drainage
	Consolidation	Lung parenchyma appearing similar to liver (hepatization)
	Pneumothorax	Absence of lung (air) sliding with respiration
Abdominal assessment	Trauma (eFAST: extended focused abdominal sonography in trauma)	Hemoperitoneum (abdominal fluid)
		Hemopericardium (fluid around heart)
		Hemopneumothorax (pleural fluid)
	Acute abdomen	Detection of abdominal collections, liver abscess, biliary pathology, appendicitis, pelvic pathologies, hydronephrosis intestinal obstruction
Musculoskeletal assessment	Pyomyositis/septic arthritis	Muscular or joint collections.
Image-guided procedures	Vascular access	Central venous catheters, Peripherally inserted central catheters (PICC)
	Guided drainage	Abdominal collections/abscess, liver abscess, pleural collections/effusion

- *Paired inspiratory and expiratory CT study*: for the dynamic evaluation of large airway in tracheobronchomalacia.
- *Contrast-enhanced CT chest*: to evaluate the lungs, mediastinum and chest wall abnormalities. Volumetric multidetector CT acquisition in most of the modern-day scanners can generate reconstructed HRCT (high-resolution CT) images, which obviates the use of traditional axial HRCT acquisition in pediatric patients.
- *CT angiography*: mainly used in vascular pathologies, congenital heart diseases.

What are the indications of imaging and appropriate imaging modality for suspected pneumonia in a child?

In suspected uncomplicated, community-acquired pneumonia in a well-appearing child who does not require hospitalization, imaging is not required.

- *Chest X-ray*
  - To document the presence, size and character of parenchymal infiltrates as well as to identify complications of pneumonia in children who do not respond to initial outpatient treatment or require hospital admission.
  - In pyrexia of unknown origin with clinical evidence of a respiratory illness and for those with fever $\geq 102°F$ or WBC count $\geq 20,000/mm^3$.
  - In suspected hospital-acquired pneumonia: new or progressive lung opacity support the diagnosis of hospital-acquired pneumonia.

- *Ultrasound*: suspected moderate or large effusion suggested by chest radiograph, should be performed for characterization, quantification and drainage, if required.

- *Contrast-enhanced CT*
  - Suspected bronchopleural fistula, to demonstrate the fistula as well as underlying causes such as necrotizing pneumonia, pulmonary abscess and empyema.
  - In suspected lung abscess, to diagnose and distinguish between lung abscess and empyema.
  - In recurrent localized pneumonia by chest radiograph (persistent opacity), to look for underlying conditions such as congenital lobar over-inflation, foreign bodies, congenital pulmonary airway malformation, sequestration.
  - In children with neutropenia, especially those after bone marrow transplant with persistent fever despite the administration of antibiotics, CECT of the chest should be considered even if the chest radiograph is negative.
  - In suspected tuberculosis, chest radiography should be done as the initial test. Lobar pneumonia with associated hilar and/or mediastinal adenopathy or cavitary air space disease is suggestive of TB. Those with equivocal finding should undergo CECT.

- *Non-contrast CT (NCCT)*: In recurrent non-localized pneumonia by chest radiograph, to look for post-infectious bronchiectasis, broncho-pulmonary dysplasia and findings such as bullae or bronchiectasis.

Imaging appearances of various pneumonia (Figure 8.1)

Viral Infection

- *Viral bronchiolitis*: bilateral interstitial opacities with peribronchial thickening and hyperinflation
- *RSV infection*: lungs are often quite clear, or focal areas of superimposed atelectasis
- *Influenza infection*: nonspecific prominence of peribronchial markings and hyperinflation
- *Adenovirus*: bronchial wall thickening, peribronchiolar densities, air trapping, and patchy or confluent consolidations. Adenopathy is more common.

Bacterial/Fungal Infection

- *Streptococcus pneumonia*: lobar/sublobar consolidation, rounded opacity
- *Staphylococcus aureus*: lobular or bronchopneumonia, pneumatoceles, pleural effusion and empyema

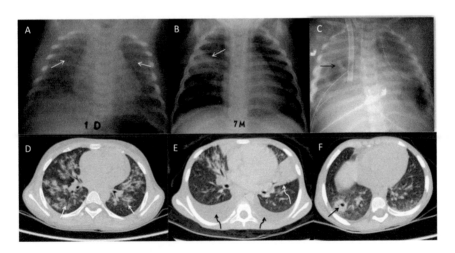

Figure 8.1 (A) Chest radiograph showing extensive bilateral reticular opacities (*arrow*) s/o viral pneumonia. (B) Sublobar consolidation in case of pneumonia in right upper zone (*arrow*). (C) Extensive right-sided consolidation with pneumatocele (*black arrow*), suggesting *Staphylococcus aureus* infection. (D) CT showing bilateral tree in bud centrilobular nodules (*arrow*) in tubercular infection. (E) Lobar consolidation (*curved white arrow*) with bilateral pleural effusion (*curved black arrow*). (F) Cavitatory lesion in case of fungal infection (*black arrow*).

- *Pertussis*: opacities surrounding heart contour (shaggy heart appearance)
- *Pseudomonas*: extensive bilateral parenchymal consolidation, patchy areas of disease with small abscess formation, or small regions of lobular emphysema
- *Anaerobic organisms*: lung abscess and necrotizing pneumonia
- *TB*: hilar and peritracheal lymphadenopathy, consolidations, cavitations, centrilobular nodules (tree in bud pattern), pleural effusion/empyema
- *Aspergillosis*: fungal ball in pre-existing cavity, nodules with surrounding halo, *air crescent sign* (air collection that partially outlines a mass-like lesion), dilated bronchi filled with inspissated mucus often cause a homogeneous branching opacity referred to as the *finger-in-glove sign* observed in ABPA (allergic bronchopulmonary aspergillosis).

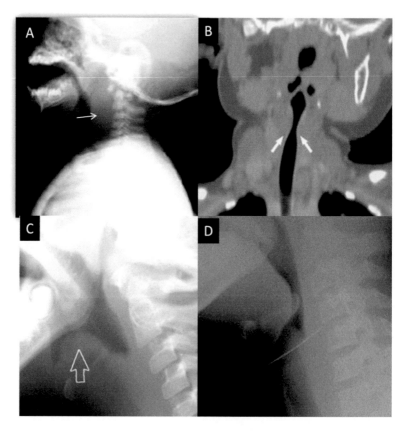

Figure 8.2 (A) Lateral radiograph of neck showing widening of prevertebral soft tissue (*arrow*), shadow suggestive of retropharyngeal abscess. (B) CT of neck shows narrowing and loss of lateral convexity (steeple sign) below the vocal cords (*arrow*) in case of croup. (C) Epiglottitis: swelling and marked enlargement of the epiglottis (*arrow*, thumb sign). (D) Linear opacity in the larynx revealing foreign body.

Child with shortness of breath

Lung infection is one of the most common causes, and chest radiograph is the primary imaging investigation.

- *Epiglottitis* is caused by *Haemophilus influenza* in preschool children. A lateral radiograph reveals swelling and marked enlargement of the epiglottis that resembles the shape of a thumb with associated thickening of the aryepiglottic folds.
- *Viral croup* or laryngotracheobronchitis is seen in children of 6 months to 3 years of age. Neck X-ray AP view shows narrowing and loss of lateral convexity (steeple sign) below the vocal cords.
- *Retropharyngeal cellulitis/abscess* is characterized by fever, neck stiffness and dysphagia. On lateral X-ray of neck, increased thickness of the prevertebral space greater than the adjacent vertebral body width below C3 and a thickness more than half of the vertebral body width from C1 to C4 level is suggestive of retropharyngeal abscess. CT is the preferred imaging modality to confirm the diagnosis and demonstrate the size, extent and location of the pus collection from a retropharyngeal abscess.
- *Foreign body*: X-ray is useful to locate opaque foreign bodies (coins, batteries, buttons), but most foreign bodies are not seen on X-ray. On AP radiographs, coins in the esophagus are seen en face as rounded opacity, whereas coins in the trachea are seen as linear opacity. In the tracheobronchial tree, aspiration of foreign body (90% are not opaque on X-ray) can lead to unilateral hyperlucent lung (most useful sign), atelectasis, pneumonia, or bronchiectasis may develop. If a foreign body is suspected clinically, an expiratory chest radiograph always should be obtained. In doubtful cases, CT can be done, which has up to 100% sensitivity.

Pediatric cardiovascular disease

- Cardiomegaly, pulmonary vascular prominence and signs of pulmonary venous hypertension and edema can be observed on chest radiography.
- On chest X-ray, complete evaluation should include a pedantic assessment of heart size, shape and position; pulmonary vasculature; the airway and mediastinum; visceral situs; and skeletal abnormalities.
- Measurement of the cardiothoracic ratio is not useful in young children, and a lateral X-ray provides a more reliable indication of true heart size (anteroposterior dimension) separate from the thymus.
- In older children, the frontal radiograph is more useful and cardiothoracic ratio is useful.
- Increased pulmonary vascularity: an arterial dimension greater than that of the bronchus is suggestive of increased flow.
- Decreased dulmonary vascularity seen in tetralogy of Fallot, tricuspid atresia.
- Hyperinflation is a sign of congestive heart failure in infants.

ABDOMEN

Imaging modalities

X-ray: main indication of abdominal radiographs are to identify bowel obstruction, perforation and urolithiasis. Dilated bowel loops are seen in ileus or obstruction. Left-side-down decubitus and upright views are used for evaluation of free intraperitoneal air and air-fluid levels.

Fluoroscopic studies: barium swallows (esophagrams) are indicated in detecting complications of esophageal atresia repair, post-operative strictures or acute post-operative leaks, radiolucent foreign bodies such as impacted food. Barium meal with evaluation of the duodenum is needed to document normal intestinal rotation. Barium/high osmolar contrast are contraindicated in cases in which viscus perforation is suspected, and Omnipaque should be used.

Sonography is the most useful modality in the evaluation of patients with GI symptoms due to lack of ionizing radiation, lack of need for sedation and widespread availability.

Computed tomography is the most sensitive modality for evaluation of solid organ, hollow viscera and peritoneal cavity pathology. MRI is indicated in hepatobiliary and pancreatic pathologies.

What are the imaging considerations in a child with acute abdomen?

Differential diagnosis for acute abdominal pain in children is broad and includes infectious, inflammatory, musculoskeletal, traumatic, gynecologic and other etiologies.

- *Suspected appendicitis* (right iliac fossa pain/periumbilcal pain): ultrasound is the most appropriate modality for initial scan. Localized fluid collection in right iliac fossa, thickened and dilated appendix loop (>6 mm) and probe tenderness are the usual imaging findings. An equivocal/non-diagnostic should be followed up by CECT, which has very high sensitivity in diagnosis and detection of complications of appendicitis such as abscess, appendicular perforation.

- *Suspected pancreatitis* (epigastric pain)
  - In case of raised amylase/lipase and presentation < 3 days of onset of symptoms, CT will offer no diagnostic advantage, and an ultrasound should be performed to look for gallstones/dilated CBD.
  - In cases of equivocal amylase/lipase values, CECT should be done for diagnosis. Alternatively, non-contrast MRI of upper abdomen and MRCP can be performed, which gives additional benefit of diagnosing biliary stones.
  - In critically ill patients, > 3 days of presentation (high clinical scores), CECT should be done to grade the severity of pancreatitis.
  - In patients with persistent SIRS, at 7–21 days of symptoms CECT should be done/repeated to look for collections and guide drainage procedures.

- Longer than 4 weeks, CECT is indicated in cases of significant deterioration in clinical status.

- *Suspected bowel obstruction*
  - Abdominal radiography is the starting point for the imaging evaluation of suspected obstruction. Dilated small-bowel loops with air-fluid levels and paucity of gas in the colon suggest small bowel obstruction (SBO).
  - US is useful in evaluating intussusception, midgut volvulus and other causes of SBO.
  - CECT abdomen without oral contrast is the modality of choice to identify the level and cause of acute bowel obstruction. In low-grade/intermittent obstruction, oral contrast can be given.
  - One of the common causes of bowel obstruction in children is intussusception (ileocolic). On abdominal radiograph, absence of colonic gas in the ascending colon and curvilinear abrupt end of colon (crescent sign) are suggestive signs of intussusception. Ultrasound is highly sensitive in diagnosis of intussusception and identification of lead point.

- *Suspected hepatobiliary disease (right upper quadrant pain)*
  - Ultrasound (US) is the first choice of investigation for biliary symptoms and can effectively show gallstones, gall bladder wall thickening or edema, pericholecystic fluid) (cholecystitis), dilatation of intrahepatic and extrahepatic bile ducts (extrahepatic biliary duct obstruction). US can also identify hepatic pathologies such as liver abscesses, hepatomegaly, liver hydatid cyst, etc.
  - MR cholangiopancreaticography (MRCP) with upper abdominal MRI should be performed for detection of distal CBD stones if the proximal CBD is dilated and distal CBD is not visualized on US.
  - CECT/MRI can be used for characterizing hepatic lesions, if there is confusion between abscess and hepatic neoplasm.

- *Suspected urolithiasis (acute flank pain)*
  - A combination of US and abdominal radiograph are the best initial modalities to detect renal/ureteric calculi. US can detect renal calculus and hydroureteronephrosis (uretric obstruction) with high sensitivity. US can also identify other differentials such as acute pyelonephritis.
  - Low-dose NCCT (reduced tube current, low kvp) has the highest sensitivity for detection of urolithiasis and should be performed in equivocal cases.

ROLE OF IMAGING IN URINARY TRACT INFECTION

- In children < 6 years, US (for pyelonephritis/renal scars) with voiding cystourethrography (VCUG), also called micturating cystourethrography (MCU), should be performed to diagnose vesico-ureteric reflux.
- In children > 6 years, no imaging is usually required, however US can be performed to look for pyelonephritis (50% sensitivity). CECT is highly sensitive in detecting acute pyelonephritis.

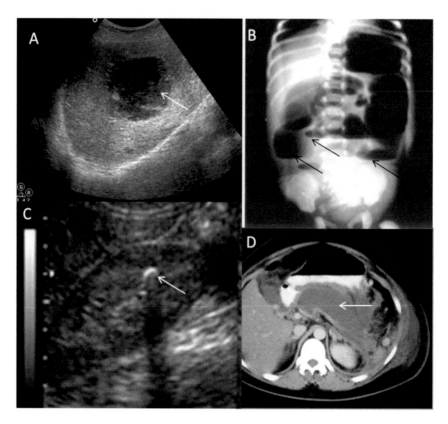

Figure 8.3 (A) Liver abscess. Ultrasound showing a hypoechoic lesion in the right lobe of liver (*arrow*). (B) Multiple air-fluid levels in the abdominal radiograph of an infant (*black arrow*) sugeestive of intestinal obstruction. (C) Renal calculus. Ultrasound of kidney showing a hyperechoic focus (*arrow*). (D) Acute pancreatitis. Contrast CT of abdomen showing acute necrotic fluid collection in pancreas and peripancreatic tissue (*arrow*).

Imaging choices in abdominal trauma

- US (eFAST) should be done to detect free fluid (hemoperitoneum), hemothorax and hemopericardium.
- Multiphase CT scanning is not necessary in children who have sustained blunt trauma. Solid organ (liver, spleen, renal) injury can be detected on CECT.
- The best indicator of pancreatic injury at CT is unexplained peripancreatic fluid. The most frequent CT finding associated with bowel rupture and mesenteric injury is unexplained peritoneal fluid. Pneumoperitoneum is a definite sign of bowel injury.
- In cases of suspected urinary bladder, ureter, renal pelvic injury, such as those with pelvic fractures, delayed urographic phase (CT urography) should be done.

BONE

Suspected physical abuse

- The appropriate imaging depends upon the age, neurological and evidence of visceral thoracic or abdominopelvic injuries.
- A skeletal survey should be performed in a child < 2 years. In a child > 2 years, target radiograph should be obtained with imaging to the areas of suspected injury, if the child is able to locate pain. A complete skeletal survey should, however, be performed in a child who has unexplained cranial or abdominal injuries or fractures that are suspicious for abuse.
- Skeletal survey with NCCT head should be done in a child with neurologic signs, complex skull fracture, apnea, multiple fractures, spine trauma or facial injury.
- Skeletal survey with CT chest/abdomen/pelvis with IV contrast is indicated if there are signs of intrathoracic or intra-abdominal visceral injury (abdominal pain/distension/bruising, abnormal liver or pancreatic enzymes).
- In children < 2 years with a high clinical suspicion for abuse and a negative initial skeletal survey, a repeat limited/focused skeletal survey should be performed 2 weeks later.
- A complete skeletal survey includes: anteroposterior (AP) and lateral skull; lateral spine; AP chest; AP pelvis; AP of each femur; AP of each leg; AP of each humerus; AP of each forearm; posteroanterior of each hand; AP of each foot.
- High specificity finding to diagnose non-accidental injury are classic metaphyseal lesions (corner/bucket-handle fracture), posterior rib fracture, scapular fracture, sternal fracture, spinous process fracture, first rib fracture. Moderate specificity findings are presence of multiple fractures or fractures of differing age, spine fracture, complex skull fracture, physeal fractures of the long bones, digit fractures.

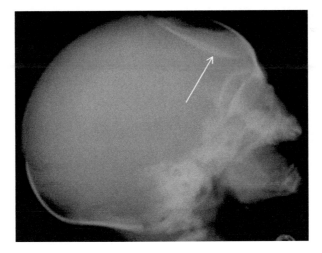

Figure 8.4 Lateral skull radiograph showing a depressed fracture (*arrow*) in frontal bone in a neonate with non-accidental trauma.

Suspected osteomyelitis or septic arthritis

- Radiography of the area of interest should be performed as an initial imaging. The earliest change on radiographs is soft tissue swelling, and the earliest bone changes are one or more small radiolucencies, usually in the metaphyseal region with or without periosteal thickening.
- MRI (modality of choice for osteomyelitis) should be performed as next imaging. T2 hyperintense area of edema can be seen in metaphysis, and eventually subperiosteal fluid and adjacent soft tissue involvement can be seen. In tubercular osteomyelitis, initial preservation of joint space, early epiphyseal/diaphyseal involvement occur with unaffected metaphysis.
- Ultrasound and guided joint fluid aspiration should be done in a child with clinical signs of septic arthritis with normal initial radiographs. Pyomyositis can be identified with US.

NEUROIMAGING

Headache in a child

- *Primary headache* (*migraine or tension headache*): imaging is not required.
- *Secondary headache*: MRI is indicated.
- *Sudden severe headache*: non-contrast CT should be done to look for subarachnoid hemorrhage. CT angiography should be performed if SAH is present, to rule out aneurysm, arteriovenous malformations.
- *Suspected brain infection*: MRI head with contrast.
- *For suspected venous sinus thrombosis*: MRI with MR venography.

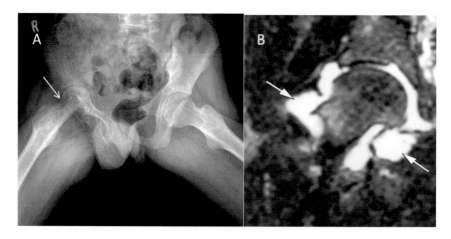

Figure 8.5 Tubercular arthritis of right hip. (A) X-ray pelvis with both hips showing ill-defined lytic lesion (*arrow*) in right proximal femoral metaphysis, (B) MRI fat-supressed T2-weighted coronal image showing significant joint effusion (*arrow*).

Blunt head trauma (PECARN criteria)

- Child below 2 years of age with normal mental status, no scalp hematoma/ palpable skull fracture, no loss of consciousness or loss of consciousness less than 5 seconds, and acting normally according to parents, no severe headache: imaging not required.
- Non-contrast CT is the modality of choice for acute/sub-acute clinically significant trauma.
- Chronic blunt head trauma with new or progressive cognitive or neurologic deficits: MRI should be done.

Spinal trauma (PECARN and NEXUS criteria)

Cervical Injury

- Low-risk cases needs no imaging. It includes absence of posterior midline cervical spine tenderness, intoxication, torticollis, substantial torso injury, focal neurological deficit, normal level of consciousness and high-risk motor vehicle crash.
- Presence of at least one of the risk factors mandates the use of radiographs of cervical spine with lateral and AP views.
- In children < 3 years, Pieretti-Vanmarcke weighted score ≥ 2–8 points, radiographs are indicated. This score was a combination of Glasgow Coma Score, Glasgow Coma Score of eye, motor vehicle crash mechanism and age.
- Traumatic spondylolisthesis at C2 or dens fractures are associated with vertebral artery injury and require CT angiography.

Acute Thoracolumbar Spine Trauma

- Radiographs to be done in all cases. NCCT/MRI may be done as a follow-up in case of abnormal radiographs.
- MRI without IV contrast has become the modality of choice.

Seizures

- In children with simple febrile seizure, imaging is not indicated. In complex febrile seizures, focal seizures, primary generalized seizures, children with intractable seizures or refractory epilepsy, MRI is usually the appropriate modality of imaging.
- The MRI epilepsy protocol should include volumetric T1-weighted imaging, T2-weighted imaging, FLAIR axial and coronal, volumetric gradient echo T1-weighted acquisitions.
- Epileptogenic lesions include malformations of cortical development, developmental tumors, anoxic-ischemic injuries, prior cerebrovascular disease (leading or focal gliosis), neurocutaneous syndromes and Rasmussen encephalitis.
- FLAIR coronal and coronal volumetric T1 should be evaluated to look for increased signal and atrophy of hippocampus to identify mesial temporal sclerosis.

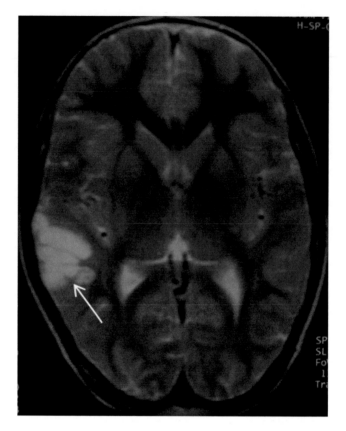

Figure 8.6 T2 hyperintese mass involving cortex of right temporal lobe suggestive of ganglioneuronal tumor.

- Tumors that can cause epilepsy are ganglioglioma, DNET (dysembryoplastic neuroepithelial tumor), pleomorphic xanthoastrocytoma, hypothalamic hamartoma.

Stroke

- NCCT head should be done in a child with clinical presentation suggestive of acute stroke. Alternatively, MRI with diffusion-weighted sequence can be performed if it is available timely.
- A child suspected of arteriopathy (e.g. Moyamoya disease, sickle cell disease, arterial dissection, vasculitis etc.) should undergo MRI with MR angiography. In children with combined features of vasculitis and hydrocephalus, tubercular vasculitis should be suspected and contrast-enhanced T1 sequence should be obtained. Moyamoya disease manifests as stenosis of terminal internal carotid arteries with collateral formation leading to a classic "puff-of-smoke" appearance on angiography.

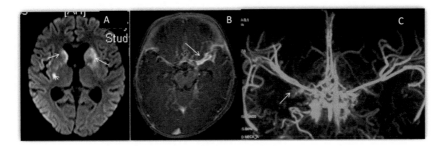

Figure 8.7 (A) Diffusion-weighted image (b1000) showing bright signal (diffusion restriction in bilateral caudate nucleus and right lentiform nucleus (*arrows*), suggesting acute infarcts. (B) Contrast-enhanced T1 image of same patient showing enhancing exudate in basal cisterns (*arrow*), suggesting tubercular meningitis. (C) Moya-Moya disease. MR angiography image showing narrowing of bilateral terminal internal carotid artery and collateral channels (*arrow*) around circle of Willis (*arrows*).

- In cases of nontraumatic intraparenchymal hemorrhage (hematoma) found on CT or MRI, a CT angiography or MR angiography should be performed to look for Arteriovenous malformation, aneurysm. In nontraumatic subarachnoid hemorrhage, NCCT followed by CT angiography should be done.
- For known or suspected high-flow abnormality (arteriovenous malformation or fistula), MRI is the preferred initial modality. MR angiography/CT angiography should be done to delineate the arterial feeders or draining vein. For low-flow anomaly such as cavernoma MRI, susceptibility weighted sequence (SWI) is recommended. MR/CT angiography is not recommended.
- For suspected cortical/dural venous thrombosis, MRI with MR venography is the preferred modality. MR/CT venography shows empty delta sign (filling defects within the sinuses).

Hydrocephalus

- Enlarged ventricles associated with increased intracranial pressure is hydrocephalus which is caused by infections, intraventricular hemorrhage, congenital anomalies such as aquaductal stenosis, venous thrombosis or tumors. Other causes of enlarged ventricles are ex-vaccuo enlargement of the ventricles as a result of volume loss.
- CT or MRI are used to assess ventricular size. Ultrasound of the head is used as the initial study in infants with macrocephaly.
- The most reliable sign of hydrocephalus is enlargement of the anterior and posterior recesses of the third ventricle. Other signs are proportionate dilation of the temporal horn along with the lateral ventricles, narrowing of the ventricular angle, widening of the frontal horn radius, periventricular edema.

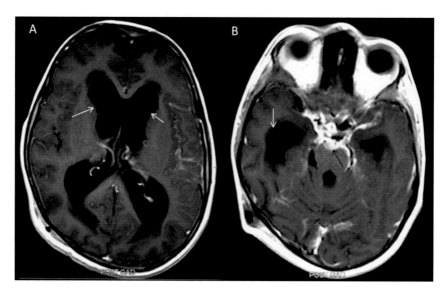

Figure 8.8 Hydrocephalus. (A) Contrast-enhanced axial T1 images showing dilated bilateral lateral ventricles. (B) Dilated temporal horns (*white arrow*) along with enhancing basal exudates (*black arrow*) suggestive of tubercular meningitis causing hydrocephalus.

Acute myelopathy

- Magnetic resonance imaging (MRI) is the gold standard examination for the evaluation of spinal cord pathologies.
- In suspected infections of the vertebral columns (Pott's spine), contrast-enhanced MRI is the study of choice, which shows involvement of vertebral body endplates and intervertebral disc subsequently extending to the vertebral bodies and adjacent soft tissues.
- In Guillain-Barré syndrome, MRI can be normal or may show thickening of the cauda equine.
- Transverse myelitis (TM) shows with increased T2 signal extending along several vertebral segments.

9

Interventional radiology in critically ill patients

RANJAN KUMAR PATEL, TANYA YADAV
AND AMAR MUKUND

Interventional radiology (IR) provides minimally invasive image-guided procedures in critically ill patients who often can't tolerate general anesthesia and surgery. Image-guided IR procedures have become the increasingly preferred standard of care in these patients with similar or improved outcomes rather than surgical intervention.

The main goals of IR in critically ill patients are:

1. Drainage of fluid collections and abscesses
2. Insertion of therapeutic or prophylactic devices (e.g. central venous line, IVC filters)
3. Control of hemorrhage (e.g. transarterial embolization, stenting)
4. Relieve obstruction (e.g. directed thrombolysis, stenting)

This chapter mainly focuses on various percutaneous image-guided drainage procedures and different types of vascular access, with a brief description about the various vascular interventional procedures in critically ill patients.

PERCUTANEOUS DRAINAGE OF FLUID COLLECTIONS AND ABSCESSES

Indication of drainage

a. Characterization of fluid that helps in modification of the antibiotic therapy accordingly

DOI: 10.1201/9781003218739-9

b. Drainage for treatment of sepsis
c. Relief of pressure symptoms caused by collection

Why percutaneous drainage, not surgery?

Critically ill patients often cannot tolerate surgery. In fact, surgery is associated with more morbidity and mortality in such patients. An image-guided percutaneous approach provides the least invasive option and is recommended in critically ill patients (*Surviving Sepsis Campaign for Management of Sepsis Guidelines*).

Role of imaging

PRE-PROCEDURAL IMAGING

- Assessment of site, size and extent of collection as well as consistency of content
- Determining the safe route of access into the abscess/collection

USG

- Easily available and less time-consuming
- Real-time guidance during the drainage procedure
- Possible to perform procedure at bedside in critically ill procedure due to its portable nature
- No radiation exposure
- Very helpful in serial follow-up without radiation exposure
- Disadvantages: poor visualization of deeper collection, anatomically difficult locations and post-operative collections (due to presence of gaseous shadow and anatomical alteration)

CT

- Provides better anatomical delineation and usually the preferred modality in difficult-to-access sites such as the mediastinum, lung parenchyma, retroperitoneum and pelvis
- Preferred in obese patients, collections with air foci and complex post-operative collections that are poorly visualized on USG
- Disadvantages: radiation exposure, time-consuming, not possible to perform bedside procedures

FLUOROSCOPY

- Usually used in combination with USG in Seldinger technique
- Used frequently for catheter upsizing and/or exchange

MRI

- A superior modality to characterize the nature and consistency of the collection
- Disadvantages: time-consuming, limited availability, need for MR-compatible devices to perform MR-guided procedures, not possible for bedside interventions, higher cost

Pre-procedure preparation

1. Coagulation profile
   - INR and total platelet count should be INR $\leq$ 1.5 and > 50000/mm^3 respectively.
   - Elevated INR and low platelet count should be corrected by administering fresh frozen plasma and platelet transfusions, respectively.
2. Prophylactic antibiotics required when draining abscess or potentially infected collection.
3. Usually performed under local anesthesia with or without conscious sedation; children and uncooperative patients may need general anesthesia.

Drainage techniques

- *Seldinger technique*: initially, access is obtained using a puncture needle (18–20G Chiba needle) followed by insertion of a guidewire. A catheter is placed within the collection after serial dilation of the tract using dilators. It is preferred in drainage of potentially deep, small, difficult-to-access, or high-risk collection.
- *Trocar technique*: a catheter mounted on a sharp trocar directly inserted into the abscess. It is better for large and superficial collections, and it is quick to perform.

FREQUENTLY ASKED QUESTIONS

Q1. Are PT/INR and total platelet counts reliable predictors of bleeding risk in every condition?

Answer: Patients with chronic liver disease have rebalanced hemostasis and the traditional coagulation parameters, such as PT/INR, and total platelet counts are not reliable to predict the bleeding risk. In addition, excessive transfusion of these blood products may increase the portal pressure and risk of bleeding, thus could be detrimental. Thromboelastography (TEG/ROTEM/SONOCLOT) allows quick assessment of entire coagulation cascade, unlike only a part of coagulation cascade by PT/INR and total platelet counts. Thus, thromboelastography is more reliable in predicting bleeding risk and should be used whenever available.

Q2. What should be done in case of thick, persistent collections and poor drain output?

Answer: Catheter exchange and/or upsizing may be required. Furthermore, instillation of fibrinolytics (t-PA, urokinase) enhances the liquefaction of debris/septations within the collection and facilitates drainage.

Q3. When should the catheter be removed?

Answer: Catheter is removed when
1. Daily drain output < 10–15 mL
2. Resolution of clinical symptoms and laboratory parameters of sepsis
3. Resolution of collection on follow-up imaging

THORACIC COLLECTIONS

a. Thoracocentesis

Diagnostic thoracocentesis

- To differentiate between transudate and exudate
- Can be performed at the bedside in a supine position under USG guidance using a 20–22G needle

Therapeutic thoracocentesis

- Indications: moderate or massive effusion causing dyspnea or chest pain
- Preferred puncture site: 6th or 7th ICS along the midaxillary line in the supine position.
- Catheter should traverse through the middle 2/3rd of the intercostal space (*to avoid injury to subcostal neurovascular bundles and irritation of the periosteum, also to avoid post-operative pain from injury of collateral intercostal nerve that passes just above the superior border of the lower rib*).
- 16G cannula or 6F catheter for single-time aspiration, 8–10F catheter for catheter drainage.
- Up to 1 litre fluid aspirated in a single setting to avoid development of re-expansion pulmonary edema.

b. Drainage of parapneumonic effusion and empyema

- Drainage required in fibrinopurulent stage of parapneumonic effusion (pleural fluid glucose < 60mg/dl or pH <7.2) and empyema.
- 10–14F catheters usually suffice.
- Instillation of fibrinolytics may facilitate drainage of complex multiloculated collections.
- Fibrinolytics are contraindicated in bronchopleural fistula.

c. Lung abscess

- Indications for percutaneous drainage: (a) Large abscess with no air-fluid levels (have high tension within); (b) no response or increase in size even after 5–7 days of antibiotics therapy; and (c) abscess in children < 7 years of age (do not drain spontaneously and less likely respond to antibiotics in children).
- Seldinger technique is the preferred method.
- 10–14 catheters usually suffice.
- Abscess should be in the gravity-dependent location during percutaneous drainage to avoid aspiration of pus into the normal lung.
- Catheter should traverse through the juxtaposed abnormal pleura into the abscess, avoiding normal lung parenchyma.

ABDOMINAL COLLECTIONS

- Shortest and safest percutaneous access route should be chosen, avoiding vital structures.

- Structures that may be traversed during diagnostic fine-needle fluid aspiration: liver, kidney, stomach and small intestine (should be avoided as far as possible during catheter drainage).
- Structures avoided during both fine-needle aspiration and catheter drainage: colon, gall bladder, and pancreas.

a. **Liver abscess**
   - Refractory and large (>5 cm) subcapsular abscesses with a high chance of rupture need catheter drainage.
   - Concomitant systemic antibiotics therapy is equally important for optimal outcome.
   - Catheter should traverse through a cuff of normal liver parenchyma into the abscess to minimize the risk of catheter dislodgment and free peritoneal spillage of purulent contents (Figure 9.1).
   - Pleura, large vascular structures, gall bladder and dilated bile ducts should not be transgressed.

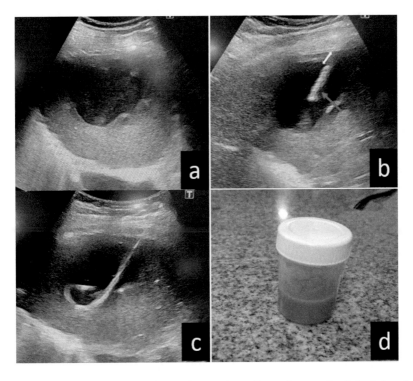

Figure 9.1 (a) USG shows a large hypoechoic liver abscess in right lobe. (b) Abscess was accessed through a rim of normal liver parenchyma (*yellow arrow*) with 18G Chiba needle (*red arrow*) under USG guidance. (c) 10F pigtail was placed over the Amplatz stiff guidewire. (d) Frank pus was aspirated from the abscess.

b. **Subphrenic collection**
  - A combination of USG and fluoroscopy is most often used.
  - CT guidance may be required.
  - Transpleural drainage may be done when no alternative safe access route is available, and normal lung parenchyma should be protected.

c. **Splenic abscess**
  - Usually occur in cases of hematogenous dissemination of infection, local spread from adjacent pathologies, and pre-existing splenic infarcts and trauma.
  - Percutaneous drainage may be considered in liquefied unilocular or bilocular collections along with broad-spectrum IV antibiotics.
  - Least amount of splenic parenchyma should be traversed during needle aspiration or drainage catheter placement.

d. **Pelvic abscess/collections**
  - Collections not amenable for drainage through transabdominal route may require transgluteal, transrectal or transvaginal approaches.
  - *Transgluteal approach*: performed under CT guidance using the Seldinger technique; catheter placement should be as close to the sacrum as possible and below the level of pyriformis to avoid injury to neurovascular bundles.
  - Transrectal and transvaginal drainage are performed using TRUS and TVS, respectively.

e. **Post-operative collections**
  - Post-surgical periods may be complicated by fluid collections (e.g. bilioma) and abscesses (e.g. leakage of bowel anastomosis, post-hernia repair abscess etc.).
  - USG guidance is often preferred.
  - Presence of air foci, post-operative ileus, anatomical alterations and superficial stitches may hamper optimal visualization of the collections/abscesses on USG, where CT guidance may be required.

f. **Pancreatitis-related collections**
  - Severe acute pancreatitis may lead to systemic inflammatory response syndrome (SIRS) and multi-organ failure, resulting in high morbidity and mortality.
  - Sterile collection is often managed conservatively with antibiotics and nutritional supports, whereas infected necrotic tissue needs removal.
  - *Indications for drainage of pancreatic fluid collections* (PFCs): (1) infected collection causing sepsis; (2) any collection causing symptoms such as abdominal pain, GOO or biliary obstruction; (3) worsening organ failure in the early phase of acute pancreatitis even without abdominal pain or any clear evidence of infection.
  - Currently, a "step-up approach" is preferred in case of an infected necrotic collection, which includes percutaneous drainage with vigorous irrigation at the beginning followed by minimally invasive necrosectomy.

- Surgical necrosectomy is often preferred at last because early surgical intervention could result in a worse prognosis compared to delayed or no surgery.

TECHNIQUES OF PERCUTANEOUS DRAINAGE

- CT is the imaging modality of choice to guide drainage of PFCs since collections are frequently retroperitoneal and associated with paralytic ileus.
- USG guidance may be used in case of large superficial collection.
- Fluoroscopy is often used to upgrade or exchange catheters.
- Preferred approach is to stay in the retroperitoneal compartment and to avoid the transperitoneal approach wherever possible; the retroperitoneal route is used later for video-assisted retroperitoneal debridement (VARD) or percutaneous endoscopic necrosectomy.
- Usual access routes: collections in or near pancreatic head and body through the gastro-colic ligament, collection in relation to pancreatic tail and distal body through the left anterior pararenal space (Figure 9.2).
- Other routes include transgastric, transhepatic and transperitoneal.
- 12–14F catheters for less viscous collections, larger catheters (14–28F) for thick viscous collections.

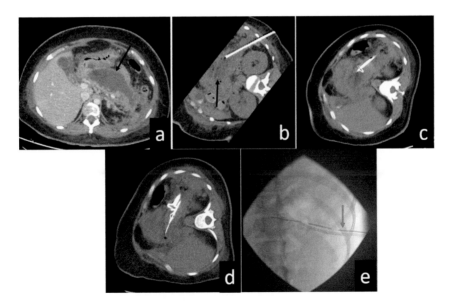

Figure 9.2 (a) Axial CECT shows a large walled-off necrosis (WON) in the anterior pararenal space (*black arrow*). (b) WON was accessed through the left pararenal approach using 18G Chiba needle under CT guidance, and (c) 16F Malecot catheter was placed. (d) Subsequently, a smaller 10F catheter was placed adjacent to 16F catheter for saline irrigation of collection, followed by catheter upgradation to 28F Abdominal Drainage Kit (ADK) catheter after few days (e).

- Catheters should be placed in the dependent part of collections.
- Multiple catheters may be required for multiloculated complex collections. Collections with thick content require frequent catheter up-gradation and saline irrigation.

Percutaneous transhepatic biliary drainage (PTBD)

Indications
- Obstructive jaundice with cholangitis, pain and severe pruritus
- Post-traumatic or iatrogenic bile leak
- To decrease bilirubin levels prior to chemotherapy commencement
- To access biliary tree for further palliative procedures such as biliary stent placement

Contraindications
- No absolute contraindications
- Relative contraindications: coagulopathy and ascites

Pre-procedural considerations
- Assessment of site and type of obstruction and selection of an appropriate target duct (right vs. left) on imaging (CT/MRI).
- Selected duct should drain at least 30% of the liver parenchyma in case of occluded biliary confluence.
- Unless infection, atrophied segment should not be drained (unlikely to improve liver function).
- Required mandatory drainage in infected biliary system due to biliary stasis; multi-segmental drainage needed when secondary confluence is involved.

Procedure
- USG-guided puncture of sectoral duct (usually segment III and VI) by an 18–22G Chiba needle at approximately 1–3 cm away from the secondary biliary confluence.
- Avoid over-injection of infected bile duct to prevent bacteremia and sepsis.
- 5F biliary manipulation advanced into the biliary tree over the guidewire under fluoroscopy guidance.
- Insertion of an 8F pigtail or 8F external-internal drainage catheter after serial dilation of the tract over the guidewire (Figure 9.3).
- Bedside PTBD may be performed under USG guidance in non-shiftable patients.
- Upon improvement of cholangitis, stricture dilatation, stenting and brush biopsy may also be performed through the existing PTBD access.

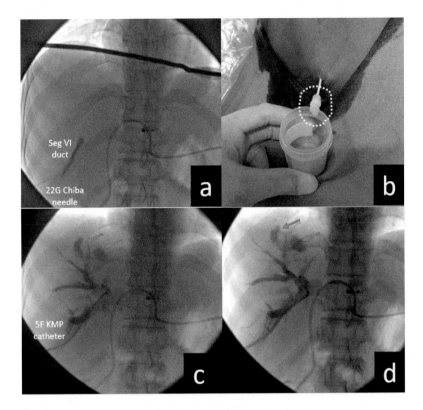

Figure 9.3   Right PTBD in unresectable hilar cholangiocarcinoma with features of cholangitis. USG showed mildly dilated right biliary radicles with multiple cholangiolar abscesses in the right lobe of liver. (a) Segment VI biliary radicle was accessed under USG guidance using micropuncture set, which showed frank purulent bile (*yellow circle*, b). (c) Access was secured by 5F KMP catheter and cholangiogram taken, which showed dilated biliary radicles communicating with cholangitic abscesses (*red arrows*, c, d). (d) An 8F external biliary drainage catheter was placed over the stiff guidewire.

Complications
- Bleeding, pericatheter leak, pseudoaneurysm formation, electrolyte imbalance and malnutrition on prolonged external drainage, catheter kinking, catheter fracture etc.

Percutaneous cholecystostomy

Indications
- Acute biliary emergencies (acute cholecystitis, acute cholangitis, or any need for biliary tract access) in critically ill patients who cannot tolerate surgery
- Relative contraindications: coagulopathy and ascites

Procedure
- Can be performed entirely under USG guidance, even at the bedside.
- Two different approaches used for access into gall bladder (GB): transhepatic or transperitoneal.

a. **Transhepatic approach**
  - 6 or 8F pigtail is placed into the gall bladder (GB) using Seldinger technique (18–22G needle) (Figure 9.4).
    - *Advantages*: greater catheter stability, reduces bile leak, leads to quicker maturation of tract (i.e. 2 weeks), and easier access in the presence of ascites
    - *Disadvantages*: higher risk of bleeding (tract traverses through hepatic parenchyma), not possible in case of diffuse metastatic liver disease

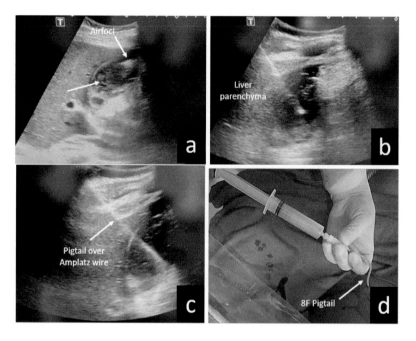

Figure 9.4 Bedside USG (a) shows dilated gall bladder with mildly thickened wall, intraluminal sludge and membrane-like structures (*yellow arrow*, a) in addition to non-dependent echogenic air foci (*white arrow*, a), s/o emphysematous cholecystitis. Urgent cholecystostomy was planned. Gall bladder wall was punctured perpendicularly through the transhepatic approach using 18G Chiba needle under USG guidance (b). (c, d) Tract was dilated over the stiff guidewire, and an 8F pigtail was placed within the GB lumen. Frank turbid pus aspirated.

b. **Transperitoneal approach**
- Trocar technique is commonly used.
  - *Advantages*: one-step process, lesser risk of bleeding (preferred in diffuse liver disease and coagulopathy).
  - *Disadvantages*: delayed tract maturation (3 weeks), higher rate of catheter dislodgement, higher risk of bile leak in case of friable GB such as emphysematous and necrotizing cholecystitis.

Percutaneous nephrostomy (PCN)

Indications
- Obstructive uropathy
- Pyonephrosis
- Urinary diversion in case of urine leak and ureteral injury

Relative contraindications: coagulopathy

Technique
- Skin entry site is usually along the posterior axillary line in the subcostal region.
- Kidney should be punctured along the posterolateral avascular plane of Brodel; lower pole calyx is preferably targeted (Figure 9.5).
- Seldinger technique is usually preferred, gross hydronephrosis with thin renal parenchyma; trocar technique may be used.
- 8F catheter usually suffice; 10/12 Fr catheter may be required in pyonephrosis.

Complications: bleeding, pseudoaneurysm formation, pericatheter leak, catheter blockage, catheter fracture etc.

Central venous access

Image-guided placement is safer, faster and with fewer complications compared to blind technique.

Indications
- Administration of IV fluids and medications, blood products, TPN and chemotherapy
- For hemodialysis, plasmapheresis and repeated blood sampling

a. **Non-tunnelled central venous catheter**
- No requirement to check coagulation profile before the procedure (lower bleeding risk procedure)
- Bedside USG-guided procedure
  - *Preferred site*: right IJV (straighter course), external jugular vein in case of bilateral thrombosed IJVs (Figure 9.6)

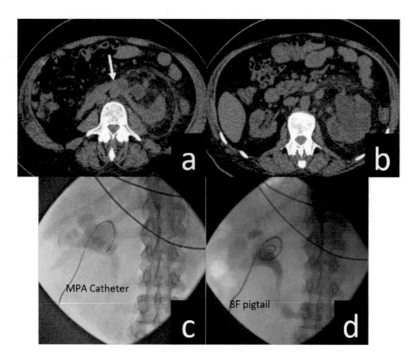

Figure 9.5 Patient presented to emergency with features of AKI and urosepsis. Axial NCCT image (a) and (b) show horseshoe kidney (communicating lower poles as marked by *yellow arrow*, a) with left pyonephrosis, as seen in form of dilated pelvicalyceal system (PCS) with marked left perirenal inflammatory stranding and fascial thickening. Urgent percutaneous nephrostomy (PCN) was planned. (c) Lower pole of left PCS was punctured under USG guidance using 18G Chiba needle, followed by insertion of a 5F MPA catheter. (d) An 8F pigtail was placed into the PCS.

- Subclavian vein is least preferred (high risk of pneumothorax and venous thrombosis).
- Post-procedure fluoroscopic spot or X-ray to confirm the position of tip of the catheter (usually 5F triple lumen catheter for adults).
- Ideal catheter tip position: SVC-right atrial junction.
- Insertion of dialysis catheter (dual or triple lumen) is same as that of central venous catheter.
- For long-term hemodialysis access, tunneled catheter in which a retention cuff is placed within the subcutaneous tunnel.

b. **PICC line**
   - *Indications*: long-term antibiotic therapy and chemotherapy.
     - It is increasingly used in critically ill patients.
   - *Advantages*: no chances of pneumothorax and hemothorax, lower rate of catheter-related bloodstream infection compared to central venous catheter.

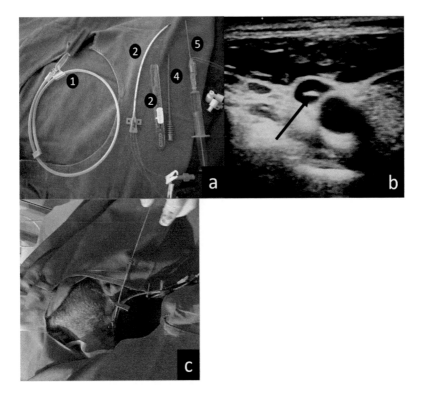

Figure 9.6 (a) Central venous line set that includes 1. guidewire; 2. 5F triple lumen catheter; 3. surgical blade; 4. dilator; 5. puncture needle with 10cc syringe (from left to right). (b) USG image of echogenic needle tip within left IJV (*black arrow*, b); (c) catheter inserted into left IJV over guidewire.

- *Preferred vein*: basilic vein > cephalic vein > brachial vein.
- *Technique*: venous access using a 21G micropuncture needle, followed by insertion of a peel-away sheath over the guidewire and advancing the PICC line through the sheath.
- *Ideal tip position*: SVC-IJV junction.
- Smallest acceptable catheter diameter is chosen to limit the development of any venous thrombosis.

b. **Arterial line**
   - *Indications*: continuous BP monitoring, frequent ABG analysis, arterial administration of drugs such as thrombolytics and use of an intra-aortic balloon pump.
   - *Contraindications*: peripheral arterial vascular diseases, anatomic variations with lack of collateral circulations (e.g. absence of ulnar artery), local synthetic grafts and local site infection.
   - USG guidance has lower complication rates.
   - Seldinger technique is used.

CONTROL OF LIFE-THREATENING HEMORRHAGE

- Image-guided endovascular embolization is preferred over surgery in critically ill patients to control life-threatening hemorrhage.
- If possible, a preliminary CT angiography should be considered: provides source and site of bleed, delineates the vascular roadmap, thereby reducing the procedure time and radiation exposure.

Gastrointestinal bleed

- Transarterial embolization (TAE) serves as an effective and safe alternative to surgical intervention for patients whose upper GI bleed is refractory to medical and endoscopic treatment.
- Coil embolization is most often preferred (Figure 9.7), occluding the both proximal and distal feeder arteries (sandwich technique).
- In acute non-variceal lower GI bleed, very super-selective embolization is needed to prevent ischemic complications.
- Microcoil, PVA, or glue may be needed as embolism materials depending upon the situation.
- In coagulopathic patients, glue rather than coil is the preferred embolizing material.
- Tumoral bleed (e.g. ruptured HCC, neuroendocrine tumor, GIST etc.) is also effectively managed by endovascular embolization in many cases.
- Transjugular intrahepatic portosystemic shunt (salvage TIPS) with or without variceal embolization (Figure 9.8) and balloon-retrograde transvenous obliteration of varices (salvage BRTO) are effective in controlling variceal GI bleed, refractory to endoscopic variceal ligation and/or sclerotherapy (Figure 9.8).

Hemoptysis

- Bronchial artery embolization is effective in control of hemoptysis.
- PVA particle is most commonly used embolizing agent for BAE.
- Coil/plug embolization may be considered in case of pulmonary artery aneurysm and arterio-venous malformation.

Traumatic hemorrhage

- Hepatic, splenic, renal and pelvic injuries are managed with TAE of bleeding arteries in case of ongoing active bleeding or prophylactic embolization in severe-grade injury to reduce the possible chance of bleeding.

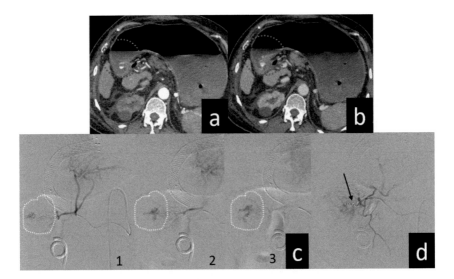

Figure 9.7 Patient of end-stage cirrhosis with portal hypertension and coagulopathy presented with massive hematemesis and hematochezia. There was profound hemodynamic instability. Arterial phase CT image (a) shows contrast luminal contrast pooling into the gastric antrum (*red circle*, a) with change in attenuation and morphology in delayed phase CT image (*red circle*, b), s/o active arterial bleed. (c) Selective angiography of common hepatic artery shows active contrast extravasation (*yellow dotted circles*) from a branch of gastroduodenal artery. (d) The concerned arterial branch was embolized with PVA particles and a microcoil (*black arrow*, d).

- Thoracic endovascular aortic repair (TEVAR) has revolutionized the management of acute aortic injury (typically type II, III injury).[1, 2] TEVAR has less morbidity and mortality compared to open surgery.
- In case of extremity arterial injuries, endovascular embolization of the source vessels or stent-graft placement may be considered depending upon the anatomical considerations (Figure 9.9).

Gynecological and obstetric-related hemorrhage

- Multiple fibroids, uterine AVM, abnormal placentation and cervical ectopic pregnancy can cause massive pervaginal bleeding.
- Bilateral uterine artery embolization using PVA, glue, or gelfoam is preferred when first-line management fails. Urgent TAE of the uterine arteries may be considered in PPH if initial managements fail as an alternative to hypogastric artery ligation and/or hysterectomy with improved survival and less morbidity.

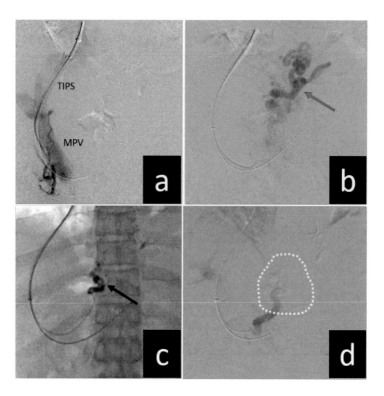

Figure 9.8 Acute esophageal variceal bleeding in a cirrhotic patient with portal hypertension which was not able to be controlled on endoscopy. (a) TIPS was created using an 8mm stent. (b) Venogram showed large tortuous lower esophageal varices, supplied by left gastric vein (LGV), which was later embolized using glue-lipiodol mixture (30%) (*black arrow*, c). (d) No residual filling was noted after embolization (*yellow circle*, d). Bleeding was controlled thereafter.

Acute vascular occlusion

- Intra-arterial thrombolysis and/or mechanical thrombectomy is a potentially salvageable option in patients with acute ischemic stroke.
- In other cases of acute vascular occlusion such as pulmonary thromboembolism, mesenteric ischemia, acute DVT, acute limb ischemia etc., endovascular interventions offer restoration of vascular patency by intravascular thrombolysis (mechanical/fibrinolytics), embolectomy and stent placement.

IVC FILTER

Indications

- *Classic indications*: documented venous thromboembolism (VTE) with absolute contraindication to anticoagulation, complication of anticoagulation resulting in cessation of therapy, or failure of anticoagulation.

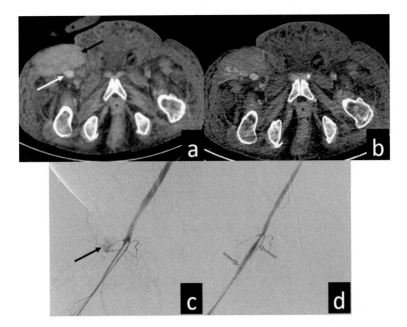

Figure 9.9 Patient having alleged history of right groin injury by a sharp object presented to emergency with hemodynamic instability and a large right groin hematoma. Portal venous phase CT image (a) shows a pseudoaneurysm (*yellow arrow, a*) just vicinity to right femoral vessels (*red circle, a*). Delayed-phase CT image (b) shows contrast jet (*red arrow, b*) into the hematoma, s/o active bleeding. (c) Catheter angiography shows contrast extravasation with a linear tract (*black arrow, c*) arising from right superficial femoral artery with diffusely narrow caliber of arteries due to hypotension. (d) It was managed by placing a covered stent of size 8 x 68 mm across the arterial rent (*red arrows, d*), following which there was no leakage of contrast.

- Prophylactic IVC filter placement is also considered in patients with medical, surgical, or traumatic conditions who are at high risk of VTE.
- *Contraindications*: complete venous thrombosis of IVC that precludes access into the IVC.
- *Types of filters*: permanent and temporary (or retrievable).
  - Temporary (or retrievable) are a newer type of filters that can be retrieved when their need is over.[3]

Technique of placement:
- The filter is deployed under fluoroscopic guidance after obtaining venous access and IVC venogram through IJV or femoral vein.
- The filter is typically deployed in the infrarenal IVC (Figure 9.10).
- Suprarenal placement is considered in cases of double IVC, pregnant patients and pre-existing infrarenal IVC thrombus.
- IVC filter can also be inserted safely at the bedside in an ICU setting wherever portable fluoroscopy is available.

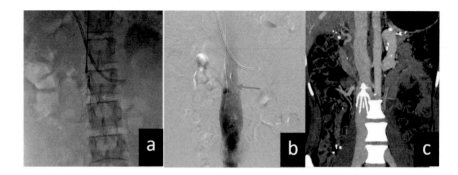

Figure 9.10 Prophylactic IVC filter placement in a 57-year-old non-ambulatory patient with rectal and gall bladder malignancy after developing right lower limb DVT. (a) IVC was accessed through the right internal jugular vein, and IVC filter was placed below the origin of renal veins after taking venogram. Post-deployment venogram (b) and follow-up CECT image (c) show infrarenal placement with passage of contrast through the filter.

ENTERAL FEEDING TUBE INSERTION

- Adequate nutritional supplementation is of utmost importance in critically ill patients, and a safe enteral route is preferred to the parenteral route when the gastrointestinal tract is functional.
- Image-guided enteral tube insertion is associated with a lower complications rate than surgical placement.
- Fluoroscopic-guided nasogastric and nasojejunal tube insertion can be considered in challenging cases when there is an obstructive pathology in the upper gut.
- Similarly, procedures such as percutaneous gastrostomy, gastrojejunostomy and jejunostomy can also be performed under fluoroscopy.

CONCLUSION

IR has changed the management paradigm in various conditions with shifting towards image-guided interventions in critically ill patients for whom surgery carries higher morbidity and mortality. Image-guided interventions also act as bridge therapy in unstable patients before definitive surgery is carried out. Therefore, IR should be an integral part of critical care units.

FURTHER READING

1. Mukund A, Rangarh P, Shasthry SM, Patidar Y, Sarin SK. Salvage balloon occluded retrograde transvenous obliteration for gastric variceal bleed in cirrhotic patients with endoscopic failure to control bleed/very early rebleed: Long-term outcomes. *J Clin Exp Hepatol.* 2020;10(5):421–8, doi: 10.1016/j.jceh.2020.04.010.

2. Sopko DR, Smith TP. Bronchial artery embolization for hemoptysis. *Semin Intervent Radiol.* 2011;28(1):48–62, doi: 10.1055/s-0031-1273940.

3. Wicky ST. Acute deep vein thrombosis and thrombolysis. *Tech Vasc Interv Radiol.* 2009;12(2):148–53, doi: 10.1053/j.tvir.2009.08.008.

4. Towbin RB, Kaye R, Bron K. Intervention in the critically ill patient. *Crit Care Clin.* 1994;10(2):437–54.

5. Mukund A, Bhardwaj K, Mohan C. Basic interventional procedures: Practice essentials. *Indian J Radiol Imaging.* 2019;29(2):182–9, doi: 10.4103/ijri.IJRI_96_19.

6. Arabi M, Gemmete JJ, Arabi Y. The role of interventional radiology in the management of hemodynamically compromised patients. *Intensive Care Med.* 2018;44(8):1334–8, doi: 10.1007/s00134-018-5236-3.

7. Rhodes A, Evans LE, Alhazzani W, et al. Surviving sepsis campaign: International guidelines for management of sepsis and septic shock: 2016. *Intensive Care Med.* 2017;43(3):304–77, doi: 10.1007/s00134-017-4683-6.

8. Dariushnia SR, Mitchell JW, Chaudry G, Hogan MJ. Society of interventional radiology quality improvement standards for image-guided percutaneous drainage and aspiration of abscesses and fluid collections. *J Vasc Interv Radiol.* 2020;31(4):662–6. e4, doi: 10.1016/j.jvir.2019.12.001.

9. Patel IJ, Rahim S, Davidson JC, et al. Society of interventional radiology consensus guidelines for the periprocedural management of thrombotic and bleeding risk in patients undergoing percutaneous image-guided interventions-part II: Recommendations: Endorsed by the Canadian association for interventional radiology and the cardiovascular and interventional radiological society of Europe. *J Vasc Interv Radiol.* 2019;30(8):1168–84.e1, doi: 10.1016/j.jvir.2019.04.017.

10. O'Leary JG, Greenberg CS, Patton HM, Caldwell SH. AGA clinical practice update: Coagulation in cirrhosis. *Gastroenterology.* 2019;157(1):34–43.e1, doi: 10.1053/j.gastro.2019.03.070.

11. Jaffe TA, Nelson RC. Image-guided percutaneous drainage: A review. *Abdom Radiol (NY).* 2016;41(4):629–36, doi: 10.1007/s00261-016-0649-3.

12. Funaki B. Catheter drainage: Seldinger technique. *Semin Intervent Radiol.* 2006;23(1):109–13, doi: 10.1055/s-2006-939846.

13. Gervais DA, Brown SD, Connolly SA, Brec SL, Harisinghani MG, Mueller PR. Percutaneous imaging-guided abdominal and pelvic abscess drainage in children. *Radiographics.* 2004;24(3):737–54, doi: 10.1148/rg.243035107.

14. Altmann ES, Crossingham I, Wilson S, Davies HR. Intra-pleural fibrinolytic therapy versus placebo, or a different fibrinolytic agent, in the treatment of adult parapneumonic effusions and empyema. *Cochrane Database Syst Rev.* 2019;2019(10):CD002312. Published 2019 Oct 30, doi: 10.1002/14651858. CD002312.pub.

15. Christensen JD, Erasmus JJ, Patz EF. Catheter drainage of intrathoracic collections. In: Kandarpa K, Machan L, Durham JD, eds. *Handbook of Interventional Radiologic Procedures.* 5th ed. Wolters Kluwer Health/Lippincott Williams & Wilkins, Philadelphia; 2016:446–52.

16. Boaz NT, Bernor RL, Meshida K, Lui F. Anatomy, thoracotomy and the collateral intercostal neurovascular bundle. In: *StatPearls.* Treasure Island (FL): StatPearls Publishing; 2020 Oct 6.

17. Klein JS, Schultz S, Heffner JE. Interventional radiology of the chest: Image-guided percutaneous drainage of pleural effusions, lung abscess, and pneumothorax. *AJR Am J Roentgenol.* 1995;164(3):581–8, doi: 10.2214/ajr.164.3.7863875.

18. Feller-Kopman D, Berkowitz D, Boiselle P, Ernst A. Large-volume thoracentesis and the risk of reexpansion pulmonary edema. *Ann Thorac Surg.* 2007;84(5):1656–61, doi: 10.1016/j.athoracsur.2007.06.038.

19. Colice GL, Curtis A, Deslauriers J, et al. Medical and surgical treatment of para-pneumonic effusions: An evidence-based guideline [published correction appears in Chest 2001 Jan;119(1):319]. *Chest.* 2000;118(4):1158–71, doi: 10.1378/chest.118.4.1158.

20. Kuhajda I, Zarogoulidis K, Tsirgogianni K, et al. Lung abscess-etiology, diag-nostic and treatment options. *Ann Transl Med.* 2015;3(13):183, doi: 10.3978/j.issn.2305-5839.2015.07.08.

21. Erasmus JJ, McAdams HP, Rossi S, Kelley MJ. Percutaneous management of intra-pulmonary air and fluid collections. *Radiol Clin North Am.* 2000;38(2):385–93, doi: 10.1016/s0033-8389(05)70169-x.

22. Wali SO. An update on the drainage of pyogenic lung abscesses. *Ann Thorac Med.* 2012;7(1):3–7, doi: 10.4103/1817-1737.91552.

23. vanSonnenberg E, D'Agostino HB, Casola G, Wittich GR, Varney RR, Harker C. Lung abscess: CT-guided drainage. *Radiology.* 1991;178(2):347–51, doi: 10.1148/radiology.178.2.1987590.

24. Charles HW. Abscess drainage. *Semin Intervent Radiol.* 2012;29(4):325–36, doi: 10.1055/s-0032-1330068.

25. Thabet A, Arellano RS. Drainage of abdominal abscesses and fluid collections. In: Kandarpa K, Machan L, Durham JD, eds. *Handbook of Interventional Radiologic Procedures.* 5th ed. Wolters Kluwer Health/Lippincott Williams & Wilkins, Philadelphia; 2016:469–77.

26. Jindal A, Pandey A, Sharma MK, et al. Management practices and predictors of outcome of liver abscess in adults: A series of 1630 patients from a liver unit. *J Clin Exp Hepatol.* 2021;11(3):312–20, doi: 10.1016/j.jceh.2020.10.002.

27. Kumar R, Ranjan A, Narayan R, Priyadarshi RN, Anand U, Shalimar. Evidence-based therapeutic dilemma in the management of uncomplicated amebic liver abscess: A systematic review and meta-analysis. *Indian J Gastroenterol.* 2019;38(6):498–508, doi: 10.1007/s12664-019-01004-y.

28. McDermott S, Levis DA, Arellano RS. Approaches to the difficult drainage and biopsy. *Semin Intervent Radiol.* 2012;29(4):256–63, doi: 10.1055/s-0032-1330059.

29. McNicholas MM, Mueller PR, Lee MJ, et al. Percutaneous drainage of subphrenic fluid collections that occur after splenectomy: Efficacy and safety of transpleu-ral versus extrapleural approach. *AJR Am J Roentgenol.* 1995;165(2):355–9, doi: 10.2214/ajr.165.2.7618556.

30. Lucey BC, Boland GW, Maher MM, Hahn PF, Gervais DA, Mueller PR. Percutaneous nonvascular splenic intervention: A 10-year review. *AJR Am J Roentgenol.* 2002;179(6):1591–6, doi: 10.2214/ajr.179.6.1791591.

31. Lahorra JM, Haaga JR, Stellato T, Flanigan T, Graham R. Safety of intracavitary uroki-nase with percutaneous abscess drainage. *AJR Am J Roentgenol.* 1993;160(1):171–4, doi: 10.2214/ajr.160.1.8416619.

32. Harisinghani MG, Gervais DA, Hahn PF, et al. CT-guided transgluteal drainage of deep pelvic abscesses: Indications, technique, procedure-related complica-tions, and clinical outcome. *Radiographics.* 2002;22(6):1353–67, doi: 10.1148/rg.226025039.

33. Butch RJ, Mueller PR, Ferrucci JT Jr, et al. Drainage of pelvic abscesses through the greater sciatic foramen. *Radiology.* 1986;158(2):487–91, doi: 10.1148/radiology.158.2.3941878.

34. Robert B, Yzet T, Regimbeau JM. Radiologic drainage of post-operative collections and abscesses. *J Visc Surg*. 2013;150(3 Suppl):S11–S18, doi: 10.1016/j.jviscsurg.2013.05.005.

35. Working Group IAP/APA Acute Pancreatitis Guidelines. IAP/APA evidence-based guidelines for the management of acute pancreatitis. *Pancreatology*. 2013;13(4 Suppl 2):e1–e15, doi: 10.1016/j.pan.2013.07.063.

36. Mukund A, Singla N, Bhatia V, Arora A, Patidar Y, Sarin SK. Safety and efficacy of early image-guided percutaneous interventions in acute severe necrotizing pancreatitis: A single-center retrospective study. *Indian J Gastroenterol*. 2019;38(6):480–7, doi: 10.1007/s12664-019-00969-0.

37. van Santvoort HC, Besselink MG, Bakker OJ, et al. A step-up approach or open necrosectomy for necrotizing pancreatitis. *N Engl J Med*. 2010;362(16):1491–502, doi: 10.1056/NEJMoa0908821.

38. Hollemans RA, Bakker OJ, Boermeester MA, et al. Superiority of step-up approach vs open necrosectomy in long-term follow-up of patients with necrotizing pancreatitis. *Gastroenterology*. 2019;156(4):1016–26, doi: 10.1053/j.gastro.2018.10.045.

39. Bakker OJ, van Santvoort HC, van Brunschot S, et al. Endoscopic transgastric vs surgical necrosectomy for infected necrotizing pancreatitis: A randomized trial. *JAMA*. 2012;307(10):1053–61, doi: 10.1001/jama.2012.276.

40. Sharma V, Gorsi U, Gupta R, Rana SS. Percutaneous interventions in acute necrotizing pancreatitis. *Trop Gastroenterol*. 2016;37(1):4–18, doi: 10.7869/tg.314.

41. Freeman ML, Werner J, van Santvoort HC, et al. Interventions for necrotizing pancreatitis: Summary of a multidisciplinary consensus conference. *Pancreas*. 2012;41(8):1176–94, doi: 10.1097/MPA.0b013e318269c660.

42. Yadav A, Condati N, Mukund A. Percutaneous transhepatic biliary interventions. *J Clin Interv Radiol (ISVIR)*. 2018;2:27–37, doi: 10.1055/s-0038-1642105.

43. Gupta P, Maralakunte M, Rathee S, et al. Percutaneous transhepatic biliary drainage in patients at higher risk for adverse events: Experience from a tertiary care referral center. *Abdom Radiol (NY)*. 2020;45(8):2547–53, doi: 10.1007/s00261-019-02344-1.

44. Madhusudhan KS, Gamanagatti S, Srivastava DN, Gupta AK. Radiological interventions in malignant biliary obstruction. *World J Radiol*. 2016;8(5):518–29, doi: 10.4329/wjr.v8.i5.518.

45. Gupta P, Maralakunte M, Kalra N, et al. Feasibility and safety of bedside percutaneous biliary drainage in patients with severe cholangitis [published online ahead of print, 2020 Oct 23]. *Abdom Radiol (NY)*. 2020;1–5, doi: 10.1007/s00261-020-02825-8.

46. Gulaya K, Desai SS, Sato K. Percutaneous cholecystostomy: Evidence-based current clinical practice. *Semin Intervent Radiol*. 2016;33(4):291–6, doi: 10.1055/s-0036-1592326.

47. Hatjidakis AA, Karampekios S, Prassopoulos P, et al. Maturation of the tract after percutaneous cholecystostomy with regard to the access route. *Cardiovasc Intervent Radiol*. 1998;20(1):36–40.

48. Dagli M, Ramchandani P. Percutaneous nephrostomy: Technical aspects and indications. *Semin Intervent Radiol*. 2011;28(4):424–37, doi: 10.1055/s-0031-1296085.

49. Ramchandani P, Cardella JF, Grassi CJ, et al. Quality improvement guidelines for percutaneous nephrostomy. *J Vasc Interv Radiol*. 2001;12(11):1247–51, doi: 10.1016/s1051-0443(07)61546-2.

50. Brass P, Hellmich M, Kolodziej L, Schick G, Smith AF. Ultrasound guidance versus anatomical landmarks for internal jugular vein catheterization. *Cochrane Database Syst Rev*. 2015;1(1):CD006962. Published 2015 Jan 9, doi: 10.1002/14651858.CD006962.pub2.

51. Schmidt GA, Blaivas M, Conrad SA, et al. Ultrasound-guided vascular access in critical illness. *Intensive Care Med.* 2019;45(4):434–46, doi: 10.1007/s00134-019-05564-7.

52. Bodenham Chair A, Babu S, Bennett J, et al. Association of anaesthetists of great Britain and Ireland: Safe vascular access 2016 [published correction appears in Anaesthesia. 2016 Dec;71(12):1503]. *Anaesthesia.* 2016;71(5):573–85, doi: 10.1111/anae.13360.

53. Heberlein W. Principles of tunneled cuffed catheter placement. *Tech Vasc Interv Radiol.* 2011;14(4):192–7, doi: 10.1053/j.tvir.2011.05.008.

54. Govindan S, Snyder A, Flanders SA, Chopra V. Peripherally inserted central catheters in the ICU: A retrospective study of adult medical patients in 52 hospitals. *Crit Care Med.* 2018;46(12):e1136–e44, doi: 10.1097/CCM.0000000000003423.

55. Trerotola SO, Stavropoulos SW, Mondschein JI, et al. Triple-lumen peripherally inserted central catheter in patients in the critical care unit: Prospective evaluation. *Radiology.* 2010;256(1):312–20, doi: 10.1148/radiol.10091860.

56. Grove JR, Pevec WC. Venous thrombosis related to peripherally inserted central catheters. *J Vasc Interv Radiol.* 2000;11(7):837–40, doi: 10.1016/s1051-0443(07)61797-7.

57. Sverdén E, Mattsson F, Lindström D, Sondén A, Lu Y, Lagergren J. Transcatheter arterial embolization compared with surgery for uncontrolled peptic ulcer bleeding: A population-based cohort study. *Ann Surg.* 2019;269(2):304–9, doi: 10.1097/SLA.0000000000002565.

58. Artigas JM, Martí M, Soto JA, Esteban H, Pinilla I, Guillén E. Multidetector CT angiography for acute gastrointestinal bleeding: Technique and findings. *Radiographics.* 2013;33(5):1453–70, doi: 10.1148/rg.335125072.

59. Ramaswamy RS, Choi HW, Mouser HC, et al. Role of interventional radiology in the management of acute gastrointestinal bleeding. *World J Radiol.* 2014;6(4):82–92, doi: 10.4329/wjr.v6.i4.82.

60. Vaidya S, Tozer KR, Chen J. An overview of embolic agents. *Semin Intervent Radiol.* 2008;25(3):204–15, doi: 10.1055/s-0028-1085930.

61. Chen Y, Yang Y, Xu WJ, et al. Clinical application of interventional embolization in tumor-associated hemorrhage. *Ann Transl Med.* 2020;8(6):394, doi: 10.21037/atm.2020.03.69.

62. Zanetto A, Garcia-Tsao G. Management of acute variceal hemorrhage. *F1000Res.* 2019;8:F1000 Faculty Rev-966. Published 2019 June 25, doi: 10.12688/f1000research.18807.1.

63. Kuczyńska M, Pyra K, Światłowski Ł, Sobstyl J, Kuklik E, Jargiełło T. Endovascular embolisation strategies for pulmonary arteriovenous malformations. *Pol J Radiol.* 2018;83:e189–e96. Published 2018 May 9, doi: 10.5114/pjr.2018.75838.

64. Padia SA, Ingraham CR, Moriarty JM, et al. Society of interventional radiology position statement on endovascular intervention for trauma. *J Vasc Interv Radiol.* 2020;31(3):363–9.e2, doi: 10.1016/j.jvir.2019.11.012.

65. Mouawad NJ, Paulisin J, Hofmeister S, Thomas MB. Blunt thoracic aortic injury – concepts and management. *J Cardiothorac Surg.* 2020;15(1):62. Published 2020 Apr 19, doi: 10.1186/s13019-020-01101-6.

66. Liu JL, Li JY, Jiang P, et al. Literature review of peripheral vascular trauma: Is the era of intervention coming? *Chin J Traumatol.* 2020;23(1):5–9, doi: 10.1016/j.cjtee.2019.11.003.

67. Weston M, Soyer P, Barral M, et al. Role of interventional procedures in obstetrics and gynecology. *Radiol Clin North Am.* 2020;58(2):445–62, doi: 10.1016/j.rcl.2019.11.006.

68. Josephs SC. Obstetric and gynecologic emergencies: A review of indications and interventional techniques. *Semin Intervent Radiol.* 2008;25(4):337–46, doi: 10.1055/s-0028-1102992.

69. Samaniego EA, Linfante I, Dabus G. Intra-arterial thrombolysis: Tissue plasminogen activator and other thrombolytic agents. *Tech Vasc Interv Radiol.* 2012;15(1):41–6, doi: 10.1053/j.tvir.2011.12.011.

70. DeYoung E, Minocha J. Inferior vena cava filters: Guidelines, best practice, and expanding indications. *Semin Intervent Radiol.* 2016;33(2):65–70, doi: 10.1055/s-0036-1581088.

71. Kaufman JA, Barnes GD, Chaer RA, et al. Society of interventional radiology clinical practice guideline for inferior vena cava filters in the treatment of patients with venous thromboembolic disease: Developed in collaboration with the American college of cardiology, American college of chest physicians, American college of surgeons committee on trauma, American heart association, society for vascular surgery, and society for vascular medicine. *J Vasc Interv Radiol.* 2020;31(10):1529–44, doi: 10.1016/j.jvir.2020.06.014.

72. Kaufman JA, Kinney TB, Streiff MB, et al. Guidelines for the use of retrievable and convertible vena cava filters: Report from the society of interventional radiology multidisciplinary consensus conference [published correction appears in J Vasc Interv Radiol. 2017 Sep;28(9):1338]. *J Vasc Interv Radiol.* 2006;17(3):449–59, doi: 10.1097/01.rvi.0000203418-39769.0d.

73. Haley M, Christmas B, Sing RF. Bedside insertion of inferior vena cava filters by a medical intensivist: Preliminary results. *J Intensive Care Med.* 2009;24(2):144–7, doi: 10.1177/0885066608330122.

74. Seron-Arbeloa C, Zamora-Elson M, Labarta-Monzon L, Mallor-Bonet T. Enteral nutrition in critical care. *J Clin Med Res.* 2013;5(1):1–11, doi: 10.4021/jocmr1210w.

75. Itkin M, DeLegge MH, Fang JC, et al. Multidisciplinary practical guidelines for gastrointestinal access for enteral nutrition and decompression from the society of interventional radiology and American gastroenterological association (AGA) institute, with endorsement by Canadian interventional radiological association (CIRA) and cardiovascular and interventional radiological society of Europe (CIRSE). *Gastroenterology.* 2011;141(2):742–65, doi: 10.1053/j.gastro.2011.06.001.

Index

Page numbers in *italics* indicate figures and **bold** indicate tables.

A

ABC method, 81
abdominal aortic aneurysm (AAA),
    34, *118*
abdominal imaging, 116–138
    abdominal aortic aneurysm, *118*
    acute cholecystitis, 131–134,
        133–134
    acute diverticulitis, 135–136
    acute pancreatitis, 127, *128–129*
    aim of, 116
    appendicitis, 130–131, *132*
    bedside abdominal radiography, 118
    cardinal technical pointers, 122–138
    computed tomography, 120–121,
        121–122, **122**, 129
    conditions that may develop during
        ICU stay requiring, **119**
    interstitial edematous pancreatitis, 129
    interventional radiology, 174–177, *175*
    introduction to, 116, **117**
    large bowel obstruction, 124–127, *125*
    modalities of, 118–121, **119**,
        120–122, **122**
    necrotizing pancreatitis, 129–130
    pediatric, 155, 162–163, *164*
    peritoneal fluid, 122
    pneumoperitoneum, 136–138, *137*
    sigmoid volvulus, 125–126, *126*
    small bowel obstruction, 123–124, *125*
    trauma, 164

abscesses
    breast, *146*
    liver, *164*, 175, *175*
    lung, 160, 174
    pelvic, 176
    percutaneous drainage of, 171–173
    renal, 100, *103*
    retropharyngeal, 161
    skin and subcutaneous tissue, 75
    splenic, 176
acalculous cholecystitis, 133
acute cholecystitis, 131–134, *133–134*
acute cor pumonale, 40–41
acute kidney injury (AKI), 98, 105,
    182
acute myelopathy, 170
acute necrotizing pancreatitis, 127,
    128–129
acute pancreatitis, 127, *128*
    in pediatric patients, 162–163, *164*
acute renal injury, 105
acute stroke, 60–61, **62**, *63*, 168–169
acute thoracolumbar spine trauma, 167
acute vascular occlusion, 186
adnexal torsion during pregnancy, 145
air crescent sign, 160
airway narrowing, 156, 158
airway reversibility, 24
ALARA (As Low As Reasonably
    Achievable) concept, 154
Alberta Stroke Program Early CT Score
    (ASPECTS), 61

angiography, CT, 47
    pediatric, 158
angiography, MR, 49
appendicitis, 130–131, *132*
    in pediatric patients, 162
arterial injuries, 185, *187*
arthritis, *166*
ascites, 98–99
aspergillosis, 160
asthma, bronchial, 20–24
atrial septal defect, 32–33
axonotmesis, 77

B

bacterial/fungal infection and
        pneumonia, 159
Balik's formula, 5
basal ganglia, 54, 55–56, *56*
    lesions of, **66**
bedside ultrasonography, 69, 97
bedside X-ray, 69, 96–97, 118
bladder and urethral catheterization,
        106, 108
BLUE (Bedside Lung Ultrasound in
        Emergency) protocol, 17
blunt head trauma, 59, *60*, 167
bone imaging, 15, 155
    for suspected physical abuse,
        165, *165*
    tubercular arthritis, *166*
bone window, 54
"boot-shaped heart," 33
"box-shaped heart," 33
brain death, 63
brain MRI, 50–53, **51**, *52–53*
    in pediatric patients, 166
    search pattern, 54–58, *55–59*
brainstem, 54, 56–58
brain tumor, 168, *168*
breast abscess, *146*
bronchi, 9–10
bronchial artery
        embolization, 184
bronchial asthma, 20–24
bronchiectasis, 23

C

cachexia, 74
caecal volvulus, 127
Canadian C-Spine Rule, 80
cardiac arrest, 42
cardiac silhouette, 10–11
cardiomegaly, 161
cardiovascular system imaging, 28–46
    abdominal aortic aneurysm, 34
    chest radiography, 29–33, *30–33*
    computed tomography, 42–43, *43*
    coronary angiography, 44
    echocardiography, 35–39, *36–37*
    factors affecting choice of technique
        in, 28
    heart silhouette, 30–31, *31–32*
    hilar enlargement, 31
    introduction to, 28
    ischemic memory imaging, 45
    magnetic resonance imaging, 45–46
    modalities of, 28
    motion mode or M-mode, 40–42, *41*
    myocardial perfusion scintigraphy,
        44–45
    pediatric, 161
    pulmonary embolus, 31, *32*
    two-dimensional method, 40
    ultrasonography, 33–34
catheterization, bladder and urethral,
        106, 108
catheters, *see* tubes and lines
cavernous sinus, 58, *59*
cellulitis, 75, *75*
    retropharyngeal, 161
central (Rolandic) sulcus, 55
central venous catheter (CVC), 7, 29,
        181–183, *182–183*
central venous pressure, 38
cerebellum, 54, 58, *59*
cerebral hemispheres, 55
cervical spine trauma, 85–87, *86*
chest X-ray
    atrial septal defect, 32–33
    cardiovascular system imaging,
        29–33, *30–33*

central venous catheters, 29, *30*
chronic obstructive pulmonary
   disease, 24
consolidation and/or collapse, 5, 6, *21–22*
heart silhouette, 30–31, *31*
hilar enlargement, 31
pediatric, 155, 156, 158
pleural effusion, 4, *4*, *18–20*
pneumothorax, 2–3, *3*
pulmonary embolus, 31, *32*
reading, *8–9*, 8–15, *11–14*
rib fracture, 5
chronic bronchitis, 24
chronic cholecystitis, 133
chronic eosinophilic pneumonia, 23
chronic inflammatory demyelinating
   polyneuropathy, 77
chronic obstructive pulmonary disease
   (COPD), 24–27
Churg-Strauss syndrome, 23
cirrhosis, *185–186*
cisterns, brain, 56
coarctation of aorta, 33
coil embolization, 184
Collins method, 3
colon carcinoma, 125
color Doppler, 15
coma, brain death and, 63
computed tomography (CT)
   abdominal, 162, 164
   acute diverticulitis, 135–136
   acute renal injury, 105
   acute stroke, 60–61, **62**, *63*, 168–169
   appendicitis, 131
   asthma, 23–24
   cardiovascular system, 42–43, *43*
   cholecysitis, 134
   chronic obstructive pulmonary
      disease, 24–27
   contrast-enhanced, 16
   coronary angiography, 44
   emphysematous pyelonephritis, 105, *106*
   gastrointestinal system, 120–121,
      121–122, **122**
   gynaecology, 109
   head, 48, 49, **49**, *50*, 53–54, 59, *60*, 67
   hydrocephalus, 169, *170*

large bowel obstruction, 125
locomotor system, 69
multislice, 16–17
nervous system, 47–48
ovarian hyperstimulation
   syndrome, 149
pediatric, 155, 156, **156**, 158–159, 162
pelvic inflammatory disease, 109
percutaneous drainage of fluid
   collections and abscesses, 172, 177
puerperal genital hematoma, 140
rupture of haemorrhagic cyst/
   endometriotic cyst, 112
scar-related complications,
   post-partum, *145*
small bowel obstruction, 123–124,
   125, 163
spinal trauma, 82, *85*
thorax, 16, *17–22*
traumatic head injury, 59, *60*, 167
tumour rupture, 112
urogenital system, *96*, 97–98
urolithiasis, 163
uterine arteriovenous
   malformations, 143
uterine artery pseudoaneurysm, 142, *142*
uterine atony, 140
computerized radiography (CR), 15
consolidation and/or collapse, lung, 5–6,
   6, *21–22*
continuous wave (CW) Doppler, 15–16
contrast-enhanced CT (CECT), *see*
   computed tomography
coronary angiography, 44
COVID-19
   diaphragmatic muscle dysfunction
      in, 73
   peripheral nerves in, 76–77, *77*,
      87–89, *88*
critical illness polyneuropathy, 78
cyst, haemorrhagic/endometriotic, 109, 112
cystitis, *147*

D

diaphragm, reading chest X-ray of, 15
diaphragmatic muscle dysfunction, 73

diaphragmatic rupture, 6–7
digital radiography (DR), 15
digital subtraction angiography (DSA), 67
    uterine arteriovenous
        malformations, 143
Dobhoff tube (DHT), 7
Doppler ultrasonography
    renal hypoperfusion and
        dysfunction, 105
    urogenital system, 97; *see also*
        ultrasonography
dose reduction, pediatric, 154–155
duplex Doppler, 15

E

echocardiography, 35–39, *36–37*
    basic transthoracic, 35–38, *36–37*
    hemodynamic evaluation by, 38–39
ectopic pregnancy, 147, 149, *150*
"egg on string sign," 33
Eibenberger's formula, 5
emphysema, 24
emphysematous cholecystitis, 133
emphysematous pyelonephritis,
    105, *106*
endocardial cushion defects, 33
endometriotic cyst, 109, 112
endotracheal tube (ETT), 7
enteral feeding tube insertion, 188
epidural haematoma, 79–80, *80*
epiglottitis, 161
Epstein anomaly, 33

F

FALLS (Fluid Administration Limited
    by Lung) protocol, 17
FAST (focused assessment with
    sonography for trauma), 98
fever, 65–67, *66–67*
fibroids, 185
"figure of three and reverse figure of
    three," 33
finger-in-glove sign, 160
fluid and hemoperitoneum evaluation,
    98–99

fluid responsiveness, 38
fluoroscopy
    abdominal, 162
    enteral feeding tube insertion, 188
    pediatric, 155, 162
    percutaneous drainage of fluid
        collections and abscesses, 172, 177
    sniff test, 73
focused echocardiography, 35
foreign body, 161
fracture, rib, 5
frontal lobe, 55

G

ganglioneuronal tumor, 168, *168*
gastrointestinal bleed, 184, *185–186*
gastrointestinal system imaging,
    116–138
    abdominal aortic aneurysm, *118*
    acute cholecystitis, 131–134, *133–134*
    acute diverticulitis, 135–136
    acute pancreatitis, 127, *128–129*
    aim of, 116
    appendicitis, 130–131, *132*
    bedside abdominal radiography, 118
    cardinal technical pointers, 122–138
    CECT, 129
    computed tomography, 120–121,
        121–122, **122**
    conditions that may develop during
        ICU stay requiring, **119**
    interstitial edematous
        pancreatitis, 129
    introduction to, 116, **117**
    large bowel obstruction, 124–127, *125*
    modalities of, 118–121, **119**,
        120–122, **122**
    necrotizing pancreatitis, 129–130
    pediatric, 155, 162–163, *164*
    peritoneal fluid, 122
    pneumoperitoneum, 136–138, *137*
    sigmoid volvulus, 125–127, *126*
    small bowel obstruction, 123–124, *125*
Goecke's formula, 5
"gooseneck sign," 33
gray scale (B-mode), 15

guided joint fluid aspiration, 166
Guillain-Barre syndrome (GBS), 78, 79, 170
gynaecology
    common disease entities, 109–114
    interventional radiology, 185
    key indications and imaging
        modalities, 108–109
    pelvic inflammatory disease, 109,
        110–111
    rupture of haemorrhagic cyst/
        endometriotic cyst, 109, 112
    tumour rupture, 112–114, 113; see also
        urogenital system imaging

H

hematoma, 75, 76
    epidural, 79–80, 80
Haemophilus influenza, 161
hemorrhagic cyst, 109, 112
headache, 63–64, 65
    in pediatric patients, 166–167
head CT, 48, 49, **49**, 50, 53–54, 67
    in pediatric patients, 166–167
    traumatic head injury, 59, 60
head trauma, blunt, 59, 60, 167
heart enlargement, 32
heart silhouette, 30–31, 31–32
hemoptysis, 184
hemorrhage, intracerebral, 61, **63**, 64
hepatobiliary disease, 163
hilar enlargement, 31
hilar structures, 11–12
hippocampus, 59
HRCT thorax, 16
hydrocephalus, 63
    in pediatric patients, 169, 170
hypovolemic shock, 42

I

infective lesions venous thrombosis, 63
insula, 55
intercostal drain (ICD), 7
interhemispheric fissure, 55
internal capsule, brain, 55–56, 56

interstitial edematous pancreatitis, 129
interstitial syndrome, 7
interventional radiology (IR), 171–188
    abdominal collections, 174–177, 175
    acute vascular occlusion, 186
    central venous access, 181–183,
        182–183
    control of life-threatening
        hemorrhage, 184
    enteral feeding tube insertion, 188
    gastrointestinal bleed, 184, 185–186
    hemoptysis, 184
    IVC filter, 186–187, 188
    in neurological emergencies, 67
    percutaneous cholecystostomy,
        179–181, 180
    percutaneous drainage of fluid
        collections and abscesses, 171–173
    percutaneous nephrostomy, 105, 181
    percutaneous transhepatic biliary
        drainage, 178–179, 179
    techniques of percutaneous drainage,
        177, 177–178
    thoracic collections, 174
    traumatic hemorrhage, 184–185
intra-aortic balloon pump (IABP), 8
intracerebral hemorrhage, 61, **63**, 64
intraneural foreign bodies, 77
intraparenchymal hemorrhage, 61
intra-spinal nerves, 78–80, 78–80
intravenous pyelography (IVP), 97
intravenous urography, 155
ischemic memory imaging, 45
IVC filter, 186–187, 188

L

large bowel obstruction, 124–127, 125
    in pediatric patients, 163
laryngotracheobronchitis, 161
left ventricular failure, 39
leiomyomas, 147
life-threatening hemorrhage, control
    of, 184
light index, 3
liver abscess, 164, 175, 175

lobes, brain, 55
locomotor system imaging, 68–89
  aim of, 68
  bedside ultrasonography, 69
  bedside X-ray, 69
  case-based reviews, 85–89
  computed tomography, 69
  frequently asked questions on, 84–85
  introduction to, 68
  long-term muscular sequelae in ICU
    patients, 74
  magnetic resonance imaging, 69–70
  modalities of, 68–70
  in muscle pathologies, 70–74, *70–74*
  in nerve injuries/neuropathies, 76–80,
    77–80
  nerve injury due to prolonged ICU
    stay, 87–89, *88*
  in pathologies of skin and
    subcutaneous tissues, 75, *75–76*
  in spinal trauma, 80–83, *80–84*,
    85–87, *86*
lungs
  abscess in, 160, 174
  consolidation and/or collapse, 5–6, *6*,
    21–22
  reading chest X-ray of, 12–15
  shortness of breath and, 161

M

magnetic resonance imaging (MRI)
  acute diverticulitis, 136
  acute myelopathy, 170
  acute renal injury, 105
  acute stroke, 169
  appendicitis, 131
  brain, 50–53, **51**, *52–53*, 166
  cardiovascular system imaging, 45–46
  cholecystitis, 134
  chronic obstructive pulmonary
    disease, 24–27
  gynaecology, 109
  hepatobiliary disease, 163
  hydrocephalus, 169
  intracerebral hemorrhage, 61, **63**, *64*

leiomyoma, 147
locomotor system, 69–70
long-term muscular sequelae in ICU
  patients, 74
myopathies, 71
nerve injuries, 77, 87–89, *88*
nervous system, 48–49
osteomyelitis or septic arthritis, 166
ovarian hyperstimulation
  syndrome, 149
pancreatitis, 129
pelvic inflammatory disease, 109
percutaneous drainage of fluid
  collections and abscesses, 172
retained products of conception,
  140, *141*
rhabdomyolysis, 84
rupture of haemorrhagic cyst/
  endometriotic cyst, 112
search pattern, 54–58, *55–59*
spinal cord, 78–80, *78–80*
spinal trauma, 82–83, *85*, 85–87, *86*
tumour rupture, 114
urogenital system, 98
uterine arteriovenous
  malformations, 143
uterine artery pseudoaneurysm,
  142–143
magnetic resonance neurography,
  84–85
mass, brain, 63
mastitits, *146*
maximum intensity projection
  (MIP), 16
medulla, 58, *58*
midbrain, 56–57, *57, 59*
mitral stenosis, 32, *33*
M-mode, 15, 40–42, *41*
multidetector row CT (MDR-CT),
  16–17
multiplanar reconstruction
  (MPR), 16
multislice CT (MSCT), 16–17
muscle pathologies, 70–74, *70–74*
muscle wasting, 74
myelitis, 78, 79, *79*

myocardial perfusion scintigraphy
(MPS), 44–45
myopathies, 70–71, *70–74*
myositis, *70*

N

nasogastric/orogastric tube (NGT/
OGT), 7
neck X-ray, 156
necrotizing fasciitis, 75
necrotizing pancreatitis, 129–130
necrotizing pneumonia, 160
nerve compression, 77
nerve injuries/neuropathies, 76–80,
77–80
due to prolonged ICU stay,
87–89, *88*
nervous system imaging, 47–67
acute stroke, 60–61, **62**, *63*
brain death in patients of coma, 63
brain MRI, 50–53, **51**, *52–53*
computed tomography, 47–48
digital subtraction angiography
(DSA), 67
fever, 65–67, *66–67*
headache, 63–64, *65*
head CT, 48, 49, **49**, *50*, 53–54, 67
interventional radiology and, 67
intracerebral hemorrhage, 61, **63**, *64*
magnetic resonance imaging, 48–49
modalities of, 47–49
MRI search pattern, 54–58, *55–59*
pediatric, *166*, 166–170, *168–170*
ring-enhancing lesions and basal
ganglia/thalamus lesions, **66**
seizures, 64, *65*
traumatic head injury, 59, *60*
neuropraxic injury, 77
neurotmesis, 77
NEXUS low-risk criteria, 80
non-bedside imaging, 97–98
non-contrast CT, *see* computed
tomography
normal KUB (kidney ureter bladder)
radiograph, 108

O

obstructive uropathy, 99, *100*
pyelonephritis, 99–100, *101–102*
occipital lobe, 55
optical coherence tomography (OCT), 27
osteomyelitis, 166
ovarian hyperstimulation syndrome
(OHSS), 149, *151–152*

P

pancreatitis
acute, 127, *128*
-induced pseudoaneurysm, *130*
in pediatric patients, 162–163, *164*
-related collections, 176
parapneumonic effusion and
empyema, 174
parenchyma, 54
Parsonage-Turner syndrome, 78
partial anomalous venous return, 33
pediatric imaging, 154–170
abdomen, 162–164, *164*
bone, *165*, 165–166
chest and airways, 156, 158–159
in child with shortness of breath, 161
computed tomography, 155, **156**
imaging appearances of pneumonia,
159–160, *159–160*
modalities and technical
considerations in, 154–155
neuroimaging, *166*, 166–170, *168–170*
radiography, 155
trauma, 164
ultrasonography, 156, **157**
pelvic abscess, 176
pelvic inflammatory disease, 109,
110–111
percutaneous cholecystostomy,
179–181, *180*
percutaneous drainage of fluid
collections, 171–173
techniques of, *177*, 177–178
percutaneous nephrostomy (PCN),
105, 181

percutaneous transhepatic biliary drainage (PTBD), 178–179, *179*
perfusion, CT, 48
pericardial drain, 8
pericardial tamponade, 42
peripheral nerves, 76–78, *77*, 87–89, *88*
peritoneal fluid, 122
permanent pacemaker (PPM), 7
pertussis, 160
phrenic nerve injury, 6–7
physical abuse, suspected, 165, *165*
pituitary, 58
pleural effusion, *4*, 4–7, *6*, *18–20*
pneumonia, 158–159
  imaging appearances of, 159–160, *159–160*
pneumoperitoneum, 136–138, *137*
pneumothorax, 2–3, 29, *30*
polymyositis, 70–71, *70–74*
pons, 57–58
post-infectious peripheral neuropathy, 78
post-operative collections, 176
post-partum haemorrhage (PPH), 139–143, *141–142*
Pott's spine, 170
pregnant patient, 139–152
  adnexal torsion in, 145
  first trimester complications in, 147–149, *150*
  interventional radiology for, 185
  introduction to, 139
  post-partum haemorrhage in, 139–143, *141–142*
  puerperal sepsis in, 143–145
  red degeneration of leiomyoma in, 147
Pseudomonas, 160
PT/INR, 173
puerperal genital hematoma, 140
puerperal sepsis, 143–145
pulmonary artery pressure, 38–39
pulmonary edema, *20*
pulmonary embolism, 31, *32*, 41, 41–43
pulse wave (PW) Doppler, 15–16
pyelonephritis, 99–100, *101–102*
  emphysematous, 105, *106*

pyomyositis, 71, *71–72*
  in pediatric patients, 166
pyonephrosis, 100, 102, *104*

R

radiography
  abdominal, 118, 162
  acute cholecystitis, 131
  acute diverticulitis, 135
  acute pancreatitis, 127
  appendicitis, 130
  locomotor system, 69
  neck, 156
  normal KUB (kidney ureter bladder), 108
  osteomyelitis or septic arthritis, 166
  pediatric, 155, 162
  pneumoperitoneum, 136–138
  small bowel obstruction, 123
  spinal trauma, 81–82, *80–84*
  for suspected physical abuse, 165, *165*
  urogenital system, 94–95, *96–97*
  urolithiasis, 163
radiography, chest
  atrial septal defect, 32–33
  cardiovascular system imaging, 29–33, *30–33*
  central venous catheters, 29, *30*
  chronic obstructive pulmonary disease, 24
  consolidation and/or collapse, 5, *6*, 21, *21–22*
  heart silhouette, 30–31, *31*
  hilar enlargement, 31
  pleural effusion, 4, *4*, *18–20*
  pneumothorax, 2–3, *3*
  pulmonary embolus, 31, *32*
  reading, 8–9, *8–15*, *11–14*
rib fracture, 5
red degeneration of leiomyoma, 147
renal abscesses, 100, *103*
renal calculi, *94–95*, *100*, *164*
renal hypoperfusion and dysfunction, 105

respiratory system imaging, 1–27
    aim of, 1
    bronchial asthma, 20–24
    cardinal technical pointers, 2–7, *4*, *6*
    chest X-ray, 2–3, *3*, 8–9, *8–15*, *11–14*
    chronic obstructive pulmonary
        disease (COPD), 24–27
    consolidation and/or collapse, 5–6, *6*,
        21–22
    disease-based reviews, 20–27
    frequently asked questions about,
        15–20, *17–20*
    interstitial syndrome, 7
    introduction to, 1
    modalities of, 2
    pediatric, 156, 158–159
    phrenic nerve injury and/or
        diaphragmatic rupture, 6–7
    pleural effusion, *4*, 4–5, *18–20*
    pneumothorax, 2–3, *3*
    rib fracture, 5
    tubes and lines, 7–8
retained products of conception
    (RPOC), 140, *141*
retrograde (RGU) and micturating
    urethrography (MCU), 155
retropharyngeal cellulitis/abscess, 161
rhabdomyolysis, 71, 84
Rhea method, 3
rib fracture, 5
ring-enhancing lesions, **66**
rupture of hemorrhagic cyst/
    endometriotic cyst, 109, 112

S

sarcopenia, 74
scar-related complications, post-partum,
    145, *148*
"scimitar sign," 33
SCIWORA, 85
secondary muscle denervation, 77
seizures, 64, *65*
    in pediatric patients, 167–168, *168*
Seldinger technique, 173
sella, 58

sepsis, puerperal, 143–145
septic arthritis, 166
septic shock, 42
shaded surface display (SSD), 16
shock, 39
    hypovolemic, 42
    septic, 42
shortness of breath, 161
sigmoid volvulus, 125–126, *126*
skin and subcutaneous tissue
        pathologies, 75, *75–76*
small airway disease, 24
small bowel obstruction, 123–124, *125*
    in pediatric patients, 163
"snowman's sign," 33
soft tissue chest X-ray, 15
sonography, 15–16
spectral Doppler/Doppler flow velocity
        waveform, 15
spinal cord, 78–80, *78–80*
    trauma, 80–83, *82–85*, *85–87*, *86*, 167
splenic abscess, 176
stent, ureteral, 106, *107*
stroke, acute, 60–61, **62**, *63*, 168–169
subarachnoid hemorrhage (SAH), 63
subphrenic collection, 176
sylvian (lateral) fissure, 55, *59*

T

temporal lobe, 55
tentorium cerebelli, 55
tetralogy of Fallot, 33
thalamus, 55–56, *56*
    lesions of, **66**
thermometer probe, 8
thoracocenesis, 174
thrombectomy, 186
thrombolysis, 186
total anomalous pulmonary venous
        return, 33
trachea, 9–10
transarterial embolization (TAE), 184
transjugular intrahepatic portosystemic
        shunt (salvage TIPS), 184
transposition of great arteries, 33

transverse myelitis, 170
trauma
  abdominal, 164
  arterial injuries, 185, *187*
  blunt head, 167
  FAST (focused assessment with
    sonography for trauma), 98
  nerve injuries/neuropathies, 76–80,
    77–80
  spinal, 80–83, *82–85, 85–87, 86,* 167
  traumatic head injury, 59, *60*
traumatic hemorrhage, 184–185
trocar technique, 173
tuberculosis, 160
  renal and ureteric, *96*
tubes and lines
  percutaneous drainage of fluid
    collections and abscesses, 177–178
  respiratory system imaging, 7–8
  urogenital system imaging,
    105–108, *106*
tumors
  ganglioneuronal, 168, *168*
  gastrointestinal, 184
  rupture, gynaecological, 112–114, *113*

U

ulcerative colitis, *125*
ultrasonography (USG)
  abdominal, 118, 162, 164
  acute cholecystitis, 131–134
  acute diverticulitis, 135
  acute pancreatitis, 127
  acute renal injury, 105
  adnexal torsion during pregnancy, 145
  appendicitis, 130–132
  bladder and urethral
    catheterization, 108
  cardiovascular system imaging, 33–34
  consolidation and/or collapse, 6
  diaphragmatic muscle dysfunction, 73
  Doppler, 97
  ectopic pregnancy, 149, *150*
  emphysematous pyelonephritis, 105
  gastrointestinal system, 118

gynaecology, 109
hepatobiliary disease, 163
interstitial syndrome, 7
leiomyoma, 147
liver abscess, *164*
locomotor system, 69
long-term muscular sequelae in ICU
  patients, 74
mastitis/breast abscess, *146*
myositis, *70*
nerve injuries, 77
obstructive uropathy, 99
osteomyelitis or septic arthritis, 166
ovarian hyperstimulation syndrome,
  149, *151–152*
pediatric, 156, **157**, 158, 162, 164
pelvic inflammatory disease, 109
percutaneous cholecystostomy,
  179–180, *180*
percutaneous drainage of fluid
  collections and abscesses, 172, 177
phrenic nerve injury and/or
  diaphragmatic rupture, 6–7
pleural effusion, 5
pneumoperitoneum, 136–138
pneumothorax, 3
puerperal genital hematoma, 140
puerperal sepsis, 143
pyelonephritis, 99–100, *101–102*
retained products of conception,
  140, *141*
rib fracture, 5
rupture of haemorrhagic cyst/
  endometriotic cyst, 112
skin and subcutaneous tissue, 75
small bowel obstruction, 123
tumour rupture, 112
urogenital system, 97
urolithiasis, 163
uterine arteriovenous malformations,
  143, *144*
uterine artery pseudoaneurysm,
  141, *142*
uterine atony, 140
upper mediastinum, 10
ureteral stent, 106, *107*

ureteric calculi, *94–95*
  non-bedside imaging, 97–98
urinary tract infection, 163
urogenital system imaging, 93–114
  acute renal injury, 105
  aim of, 93
  bedside imaging, 96–97
  bedside ultrasonography, 97
  bladder and urethral catheterization,
    106, 108
  computed tomography, 97–98
  Doppler ultrasonography, 97
  emphysematous pyelonephritis, 105, *106*
  evaluation of fluid and
    hemoperitoneum, 98–99
  intravenous pyelography, 97
  introduction to, 93, *94–96*
  magnetic resonance imaging, 98
  modalities of, 96–98
  normal KUB (kidney ureter bladder)
    radiograph, 108
  obstructive uropathy, 99, *100*
  percutaneous nephrostomy, 105
  pyelonephritis, 99–100, *101–102*
  pyonephrosis, 100, 102, *104*
  renal hypoperfusion and
    dysfunction, 105
  tubes and catheters, 105–108, *106*

ureteral stent, 106, *107*; *see also*
  gynaecology
urolithiasis, 163
urosepsis, *182*
uterine arteriovenous malformations
  (AVMs), 143, *144*
uterine artery embolization, 185
uterine artery pseudoaneurysm,
  140–143, *143*
uterine atony, 140

V

venography
  computed tomography, 47
  magnetic resonance, 49
venous thromboembolism (VTE),
  186–187
ventilation perfusion (VQ), 2
ventricles, brain, 54, 56, 169, *170*
viral croup, 161
viral pneumonia, 159
volume rendering (VR), 16

W

wall area percent, 26
Westermark's sign, 31, *32*